SPORTS EMERGENCY CARE A Team Approach

SPORTS EMERGENCY CARE A Team Approach

Robb S. Rehberg, PhD, ATC, CSCS, NREMT
Assistant Professor and
Coordinator of Athletic Training Clinical Education
William Paterson University
Wayne, NJ
Director of Emergency Services
Montclair State University
Montclair, NJ

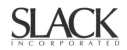

Delivering the best in health care information
and education worldwide

RC
1210
.S6754
2007

ISBN: 978-1-55642-798-5
Copyright © 2007 by SLACK Incorporated

Sports Emergency Care: A Team Approach Instructor's Manual is also available from SLACK Incorporated. Don't miss this important companion to *Sports Emergency Care: A Team Approach.* To obtain the Instructor's Manual, please visit http://www.efacultylounge.com.

All photos, unless otherwise credited, appear courtesy of Robb S. Rehberg.

The procedures and practices described in this book should be implemented in a manner consistent with the professional standards set for the circumstances that apply in each specific situation. Every effort has been made to confirm the accuracy of the information presented and to correctly relate generally accepted practices. The authors, editor, and publisher cannot accept responsibility for errors or exclusions or for the outcome of the material presented herein. There is no expressed or implied warranty of this book or information imparted by it. Care has been taken to ensure that drug selection and dosages are in accordance with currently accepted/recommended practice. Due to continuing research, changes in government policy and regulations, and various effects of drug reactions and interactions, it is recommended that the reader carefully review all materials and literature provided for each drug, especially those that are new or not frequently used. Any review or mention of specific companies or products is not intended as an endorsement by the author or publisher.

SLACK Incorporated uses a review process to evaluate submitted material. Prior to publication, educators or clinicians provide important feedback on the content that we publish. We welcome feedback on this work.

Contact SLACK Incorporated for more information about other books in this field or about the availability of our books from distributors outside the United States.

Published by: SLACK Incorporated
6900 Grove Road
Thorofare, NJ 08086 USA
Telephone: 856-848-1000
Fax: 856-853-5991
www.slackbooks.com

Sports emergency care : a team approach / [edited by] Robb S. Rehberg.
    p. ; cm.
Includes bibliographical references and index.
ISBN 978-1-55642-798-5 (alk. paper)
1. Sports emergencies. 2. Sports medicine. 3. Sports injuries--Treatment. I. Rehberg, Robb S.
[DNLM: 1. Athletic Injuries--therapy. 2. Emergency Treatment. QT 261 S7639 2007]
RC1210.S6754 2007
617.1'027--dc22
                                                2007007887

For permission to reprint material in another publication, contact SLACK Incorporated. Authorization to photocopy items for internal, personal, or academic use is granted by SLACK Incorporated provided that the appropriate fee is paid directly to Copyright Clearance Center. Prior to photocopying items, please contact the Copyright Clearance Center at 222 Rosewood Drive, Danvers, MA 01923 USA; phone: 978-750-8400; website: www.copyright.com; email: info@copyright.com

Printed in the United States of America.

Last digit is print number: 10 9 8 7 6 5 4 3 2

Dedication

For my beautiful wife, Joelle, for her love, encouragement, and patience.
This project would not have been possible without you;

For my wonderful children, Anna and Joseph, for their unending supply
of hugs and kisses and for never letting me forget what is most important in
life;

For my parents, who always told me that I could do anything if I put my
mind to it;

For my colleagues, the athletic trainers and EMTs who, day in and day
out, selflessly help others in need. You are the inspiration for this book.

Contents

Acknowledgments

Developing *Sports Emergency Care: A Team Approach* was just that ... a team approach. There are several people who were instrumental in the development of this book that I wish to thank. Without their help, this book would never have been written.

To the contributing authors:

Mike Cendoma, who has spent his career researching and teaching others how to prepare for sports emergencies. I admire your dedication to educating others, and I thank you for contributing your work on management of spinal injuries and mild traumatic brain injury to this book. I am honored to have you as part of the team.

Mike Prybicien, my colleague and longtime friend. We have come a long way from those early days in our careers. Thanks for being involved in this project and for helping out in so many ways.

John Davis (the "cover boy" for the book), you are a friend, colleague, and role model. It meant a lot to have you involved in this project. Thanks for everything.

Jeff Konin, I am honored to have you involved in this project. Thanks for your contribution to this book, as well as for your mentorship and friendship. You make this stuff look easy.

Dave Middlemas, this book is better because of your involvement. Thanks for your contribution, your friendship, and also for your help with the photo shoot.

Lou Rizio, for finding the time in your busy schedule to contribute to this project. Your contributions were invaluable.

Joelle Rehberg, for illustrating much of the line art that appears in this book, countless hours of manuscript review, and simply for putting up with me in the process.

Thanks also to the athletic training faculty and staff at William Paterson University: Linda Gazzillo Diaz, Toby Barboza, Dondi Boyd, and Jaclyn Norberg, for their never-ending assistance in getting this book off the ground. Thanks also to the athletic training students of William Paterson University, especially Matthew Bergh and Tedd Rossillo (who served as models), and the athletic training students and EMS staff at Montclair State University for participating in the photo shoot for this book.

Special thanks to the staff at SLACK Incorporated, especially Jennifer Briggs, Kim Shigo, April Billick, and especially to Carrie Kotlar for believing in this book and finally making it happen.

About the Author

Robb S. Rehberg, PhD, ATC, CSCS, NREMT is an Assistant Professor and Coordinator of Athletic Training Clinical Education at William Paterson University in Wayne, NJ. He also serves as the Director of Emergency Services at Montclair State University in Montclair, NJ. Prior to teaching at William Paterson, Dr. Rehberg spent 13 years as the head athletic trainer at Westwood Regional High School in Westwood, NJ. Dr. Rehberg earned his PhD in Health Science from Touro University International in 2003, a Master's of Sport Science degree from the United States Sports Academy in 1999, and a Bachelor's of Science in Athletic Training from West Chester University in 1991.

Dr. Rehberg has spent his career working in both the athletic training and emergency services fields and has published and spoken frequently at state and national meetings on sports emergency care. Dr. Rehberg served as a member of the medical staff for athletics (track and field) at the 1996 Olympic Games in Atlanta, Ga. He has been active on the state and national level, having served on the National Athletic Trainers' Association (NATA) Inter-Association Task Force for the Appropriate Care of the Spine-Injured Athlete, the Task Force on Appropriate Medical Coverage for the Secondary School-Aged Athlete, and the NATA Hall of Fame Subcommittee. Dr. Rehberg currently serves as President of the Athletic Trainers' Society of New Jersey. He has also served as the Chair of the National Safety Council Emergency Care Advisory Committee since 1992 and was a member of the American Heart Association Task Force that developed the first-ever international guidelines for first aid in 2000. He is a charter member of the New Jersey Disaster Medical Assistance Team.

Contributing Authors

Michael J. Cendoma, MS, ATC
Director
Sports Medicine Concepts
Geneseo, NY

John L. Davis, MS, ATC
Coordinator of Athletic Training and Sports Medicine Services
Montclair State University
Montclair, NJ

Jeff G. Konin, PhD, ATC, PT
Associate Professor
Department of Orthopaedic Surgery
Executive Director
Sports Medicine & Athletic Related Trauma (SMART) Institute
College of Medicine
University of South Florida
Tampa, Fla

David A. Middlemas, EdD, ATC
Director
Athletic Training Education Program
Montclair State University
Montclair, NJ

Michael Prybicien, MA, ATC, EMT-B, CSCS
Head Athletic Trainer
Passaic High School
Passaic, NJ

Louis Rizio III, MD
Director of Sports Medicine
Sports Medicine and Orthopaedic Center
Livingston, NJ

Preface

There have been illnesses and injuries related to sports for as long as there have been organized sports. Some of these conditions can be life and limb threatening and are considered emergencies. While life-threatening injuries and illnesses do not occur often, proper management of these conditions is arguably the most important job that members of the sports emergency care team will ever face.

Sports Emergency Care: A Team Approach was primarily designed to fill the void that has traditionally existed in athletic training education on the subject of emergency care. Traditionally, athletic training educators have had to resort to developing courses based on existing first aid materials or developing materials on their own in order to meet the needs of the athletic training student. This book contains all the necessary information needed to prepare athletic training students beyond traditional first aid training.

This book was also designed to provide specific information on emergency situations in sports for emergency medical services (EMS) professionals. To date, no such text has ever addressed sports emergency care for EMS providers. While this book was written with athletic trainers, athletic training students, and EMS personnel in mind, all health care providers who play a role on the sports emergency care team will find this book useful in preparing for emergency situations in sports.

This book can be used in several different ways. It can be used in athletic training education programs as a core textbook as part of a sports emergency care course. It can also be used as a supplemental text in several courses that address immediate care within an athletic training education curriculum. EMS educators may also find this book useful in developing continuing education programs for prehospital providers. An added feature that instructors will find helpful is the *Sports Emergency Care: A Team Approach Instructor's Manual*, which was developed to guide instructors in the delivery of course content. Complete with lecture outlines, test questions, and lab activities, the instructor manual is a valuable tool that can be used in developing a sports emergency care course.

Finally, this book is also designed to be used as a reference and field guide for all health care providers who serve as members of the sports emergency care team, including athletic trainers, emergency medical technicians and paramedics, and physicians.

Regardless of discipline, it is important for all health care providers charged with caring for ill or injured athletes to be knowledgeable and proficient in managing sports emergencies. This ability can only be achieved through preparation and practice. Health care providers who utilize this book to enhance their emergency care skills and practice together as a team will ultimately be prepared to provide the best care possible in emergency situations.

Foreword

Although most injuries in athletics are relatively minor, life- or limb-threatening injuries are unpredictable and can occur without warning. Due to the relatively low incidence rate of catastrophic injuries, health care providers may develop a false sense of security. Catastrophic injuries can occur during any physical activity and at any level of participation. When this happens, there is typically heightened public awareness associated with the nature and management of the emergency situation. Medical-legal interests may lead to questions regarding qualifications of the health care personnel involved, the preparedness of the athletic organization, and actions taken.

In an emergency situation, proper management of life- and limb-threatening injuries is critical. Ideally, properly trained medical and allied health personnel should handle emergencies. Preparation should include education and training in emergency evaluation and management of injuries and illnesses, emergency procedures, selection and maintenance of emergency equipment and supplies, appropriate use of emergency personnel, and formation and implementation of an emergency action plan.

Emergencies are rarely predictable. When they occur, a rapid but controlled response is indicated. All personnel involved with the organization or sponsorship of athletic activities share a professional responsibility to provide for the emergency care of an injured person. The goal of the sports medicine team is delivery of the highest possible quality of health care to the athlete. Accordingly, the sports medicine team must work together as an efficient unit to accomplish these goals. By sharing information, training, and skills between team members, the injured or ill athlete may receive the highest quality emergency care. The importance of being prepared when emergencies occur cannot be stressed enough. Survival may hinge on how well trained and prepared athletic health care providers are.

Sports Emergency Care: A Team Approach is a valuable educational tool in the area of athletic emergencies. By reading and reviewing in the area of emergency medicine, the health care provider better prepares to manage athletic emergencies. Vince Dooley, head football coach for the University of Georgia, was often quoted as saying, "Proper preparation prevents poor performance." This is particularly true in the area of emergency medicine. Be well prepared in all of your endeavors!

Ron Courson, ATC, PT, NREMT-I, CSCS
Director of Sports Medicine
University of Georgia
Athens, Ga

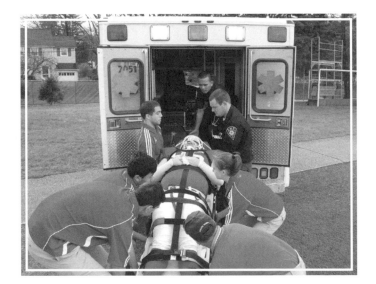

Introduction to Sports Emergency Care

Chapter 1

Robb S. Rehberg, PhD, ATC, CSCS, NREMT

A 14-year-old male high school cross country athlete suddenly collapses after finishing a 5-mile practice run...
A 14-year-old female high school basketball player collapses on the bench during a game...
An 18-year-old high school wrestler injures his neck during a match. He cannot move his arms or legs...
A high school baseball player is hit in the neck by a line drive-batted ball while pitching batting practice. The athlete collapses and is unconscious...
An 18-year-old male track athlete was impaled by a javelin during track practice...
A high school football player is injured during a game after tackling with his head down, resulting in helmet-to-helmet contact. He lies motionless on the turf.

These types of emergencies occur every season on the courts and fields; at the professional, college, high school, and youth levels; and in organized and informal activities. *Are you prepared to handle these emergencies?*

Health care professionals who are entrusted with the health and safety of athletes must ask themselves this question every day. The possibility of serious injury or sudden illness exists in all sports, regardless of the level or type of play. The examples above are based on real situations in which an athlete died or became permanently disabled.[1] It is not enough for health care professionals to renew their cardiopulmonary resuscitation (CPR) certification every 2 years and hope for the best. Health care professionals who work with athletes must have a unique understanding of the potential emergency situations that can arise and must posses the skills and knowledge to manage such emergencies. They must be proficient in sports emergency care.

What Is Sports Emergency Care?

Emergency care is defined as the immediate care given to an injured or suddenly ill person. Practitioners of emergency care must be proficient in the recognition of sudden illness and injury, as well as possess skills necessary to manage the condition until more definitive medical care is available. Emergency care usually goes beyond first aid treatment and may involve more advanced skills and specialized equipment. Keeping this definition in mind, sports emergency care can be defined as the immediate care given to an injured or suddenly ill sports participant. Sports emergency care is an area of specialization that is necessary for health care providers who are involved in caring for physically active individuals.

Why Is Sports Emergency Care Needed?

There is an inherent risk of injury in sports. In more physically demanding sports, athletes compete at full speed, with great intensity, and in some cases, at the expense of bodily injury. While the incidence of catastrophic injury in sports is relatively low, immediate recognition of emergencies and appropriate care is crucial in order to provide the athlete with the best chance of survival. Health care professionals covering sports must be prepared for injuries and illnesses that are a direct result of sports participation (such as spinal injuries, head injuries, and fractures), as well as indirect causes (such as congenital heart abnormalities and other medical emergencies). The needs of sports participants with these types of injuries and illnesses go far beyond first aid care. Specialized knowledge of such situations and their unique relationship to sports participation are necessary to provide the best care possible.

Sports Emergency Care: A Team Approach

Preparing for and managing sports emergencies must be a team effort. Each member of the team must understand, respect, and appreciate the capabilities and specialized skills possessed by the other members of the team. Historically, there have been situations in which athletic trainers and emergency medical technicians (EMTs) have differed in their approach to managing emergency situations in sports (the issue of athletic helmet removal has traditionally been at the center of this controversy). Oftentimes, this difference in approach can lead to on-field confrontation at the scene of an emergency. It is not hard to see why athletic trainers and EMTs may, at times, differ in their approach to managing a specific injury or illness. After all, the background, training, and areas of specialization differ for each discipline. However, prior planning and dialogue among all health care professionals involved in managing sports emergencies can yield a competent sports emergency care team that is prepared to work efficiently together.

The sports emergency care team is a subset of the sports medicine team that includes individuals with specialized training in emergency care. Naturally, the athletic trainer will be a key player in the sports emergency care team. Other important members of the team include, but are not limited to, EMTs and paramedics, medical first responders, emergency nurses, and physicians. The sports emergency care team should highlight each member's strengths. For instance, EMTs may have more experience in the packaging of cervical-spine injuries than any other team member. Conversely, the athletic trainer may be more familiar with the equipment worn by the athlete (ie, helmet, shoulder pads) and have a deeper knowledge of neurological function and assessment. The physician, if present, may have an even deeper understanding of the pathophysiology of the injury and possible complications. Understanding the strengths of each team member and learning how to best put each team member's strengths to use comes only through practice and is essential for providing quality emergency care to the injured athlete.

How to Use This Book

It is the author's vision that members of the sports emergency care team—athletic trainers, EMTs, physicians, and others—will utilize this book to further their knowledge and skills in the management of sports emergencies. However, just reading this text is not enough. Sports emergency care must be a team approach. Health care professionals must practice together often to refine skills, stimulate discussion, foster teamwork, and identify deficiencies in the emergency plan. Ultimately, patient care in the field relies on sound judgment, planning, and teamwork.

In addition to practicing sports emergency care, all members of the sports emergency care team should maintain current certification in CPR at the professional rescuer level, in addition to maintaining continuing education requirements necessary to maintain their respective credentials.

There may be skills and techniques presented in this book that fall outside the scope of practice for some health care professionals. Readers should always act within their scope of practice. Moreover, local protocols may differ from information presented. Sports emergency care personnel should always follow local protocol.

ATHLETIC TRAINERS

In most cases, it is the athletic trainer who will be at the center of the sports emergency care team. Athletic trainers have a strong background in anatomy and physiology and extensive knowledge of athletic injuries and illnesses. However, while athletic trainers routinely handle musculoskeletal injuries and other conditions, they rarely handle emergencies. Therefore, it is important for athletic trainers, regardless of the setting, to develop a sports emergency care team to ensure the proper care for the athletes they serve. The information contained in this book will provide the athletic trainer with a deeper understanding of the types of emergencies that can occur in sports. However, athletic trainers are urged to strive to learn as much as possible about emergency care and the emergency medical services (EMS) system that responds to their place of employment. Athletic trainers might consider riding along with the local EMS unit to gain a better understanding of the EMS system and the training and background of EMTs and paramedics. Athletic trainers may also consider enrolling in an EMT or medical first responder course to increase their depth of knowledge of emergency care.

EMS Personnel

The EMT-Basic National Standard Curriculum, from which EMT training is based, provides a foundation for the management of a number of medical and trauma situations. However, EMT training cannot and does not cover every conceivable emergency. While EMTs handle medical emergencies more frequently than athletic trainers, most EMTs are largely unfamiliar with the unique nature of sports injury and illness, mechanisms of sports injury, and equipment used in certain sports. It is important for the practicing EMT to seek continuing education to strengthen his or her knowledge in areas in which he or she will ultimately find him- or herself involved. There are a number of continuing education programs available for EMTs, from hazardous materials to incident command. EMTs who are involved in the coverage of sporting events should be familiar with the types of illness and injury germane to the sports environment, as well as an understanding of mechanism of injury, equipment used, and unique situations that can present in an emergency. EMTs should also consider working with a local athletic trainer and observing day-to-day activities in order to obtain a better understanding of athletic injuries and illnesses, as well as a better appreciation of the field of athletic training.

Educators

Athletic training education programs have undergone a major transformation in the past decade. Clinical proficiencies and competencies on immediate care of athletic injury and illness are a critical part of an athletic training student's education. However, content on sports emergencies is often piecemeal, and courses used to cover immediate care competencies and proficiencies usually consist of first aid courses being "retrofitted" to cover emergencies. However, sports emergency care goes beyond typical first aid training. This text can be used in athletic training education programs as a stand-alone course or in several athletic training courses to cover information in the immediate care of sports emergencies. Athletic training educators are also encouraged to involve the local EMS agencies in their education program to further strengthen the bond between athletic training and EMS.

EMS educators may want to consider developing a continuing education course focusing on sports emergency care. Specialized continuing education training programs are widely available on topics such as trauma, pediatrics, geriatrics, and farm injuries. The types of injuries and illnesses related to sports participation also warrant specialized education, especially for those EMS professionals who cover sporting events. EMS educators could benefit from collaborating with athletic trainers in the development and implementation of such programs.

Train. Often. Together. The athletes you serve are depending on you.

References

1. Mueller FO, Cantu RC. National Center for Catastrophic Sports Injury Research: twenty-third annual report: fall 1982–spring 2005. Available at: http://www.unc.edu/depts/nccsi/AllSport.htm. Accessed November 15, 2006.

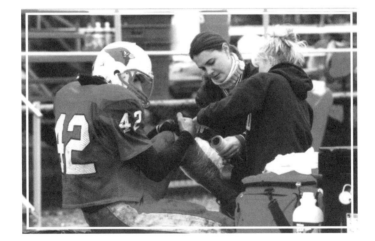

Chapter 2

Preparing for Sports Emergencies

Robb S. Rehberg, PhD, ATC, CSCS, NREMT

Proper management of emergencies in sports does not happen by accident. Preparation is the key to ensuring that the appropriate resources and procedures exist to ensure the best care possible. Preparation for sports emergencies is a dynamic process, and planning should begin well in advance of the injury, game, or even the season.

There are many factors that should be considered when preparing for sports emergencies. In order to address each of these factors, the acronym PREPARE can be used. PREPARE emphasizes the critical elements of emergency planning: Personnel, Rules, Equipment, Planning, Arena, Rehearsal, and Evaluate and Educate. Each of these critical elements must be addressed when developing an emergency action plan (EAP) for sports emergencies.

Personnel

Who are the members of your sports emergency care team? This question may be answered differently depending on the level of play and the size of the institution. A sports emergency care team in the National Football League may have more members than a small high school. All personnel must be identified and included in the preparation and planning process regardless of the size of the venue or the number of members of the team. It is important that each member of the team understands the qualifications, expertise, and limitations of the other members. It is equally important for all team members to be comfortable with the capabilities and roles of each team member. Some of the personnel that should be included in the sports emergency care team include athletic trainers, EMS personnel, physicians, hospital staff, coaching staff, athletic training students, athletics staff, athletes, and other personnel.

ATHLETIC TRAINERS

Certified athletic trainers are medical professionals who are experts in injury prevention, assessment, treatment, and rehabilitation, particularly in the orthopedic and musculoskeletal disciplines. Athletic trainers have been recognized by the American Medical Association as allied health care professionals since 1990. In order to be eligible for board certification, athletic trainers must graduate from an accredited undergraduate or graduate athletic training curriculum, which consists of course work and clinical experience in several areas, including assessment and evaluation, acute care, general medical conditions and disabilities, and pathology of injury and illness. Athletic trainers must hold a minimum of a bachelor's degree, although nearly three-quarters of all certified athletic trainers hold a master's degree or higher. In addition to board certification, many states regulate the athletic training profession through licensure, registration, or certification.

In most situations, the athletic trainer will be the "captain" of the sports medicine team. The athletic trainer is often responsible for assembling the sports emergency care team, developing site-specific EAPs, ordering necessary equipment, ensuring that the members of the team are informed of the plan, and conducting regular training and drills.

EMERGENCY MEDICAL SERVICES PERSONNEL

EMS personnel are important members of the sports emergency care team. Ultimately, it will be the EMS personnel who will assume responsibility for packaging and transporting the injured athlete to the hospital. There are 3 distinct levels of emergency care providers: first responders, EMTs, and paramedics. Each level of training represents a different level of expertise in the continuum of emergency medical care. EMS education follows a national standard curriculum established by the National Highway Traffic Safety Administration's Emergency Medical Services Program. First responders are the most basic level of EMS training. First responders are trained to assess and stabilize ill and injured patients until additional EMS assistance arrives. First responders complete approximately 40 hours of training in the areas of assessment, airway management, management of medical and trauma emergencies, and emergency childbirth. Police officers, firefighters, and lifeguards are often trained at the first responder level.

EMTs are the next level in the continuum of EMS training. EMT-Basics (also known in some states as EMT-B, EMT-1, EMT-A, or EMT-D) undergo approximately 110 hours to 120 hours of EMS training in patient assessment, airway management, management of respiratory and cardiac emergencies, management of medical and trauma emergencies, bleeding, fractures, and emergency childbirth. EMTs can usually administer or assist in the administration of oxygen, epinephrine (for allergic reactions), nitroglycerine, and metered dose inhalers depending on state or local protocols. EMT-Intermediates (EMT-I) require a higher level of training (approximately 200 hours to 400 hours). EMT-Intermediates can perform all the functions of an EMT-Basic and can also administer intravenous fluids and certain medications, depending on state or local protocol. EMT-Paramedic (EMT-P) is the highest level of EMS training, consisting of over 1000 hours of training. EMT-Paramedics can perform advanced procedures and administer a wider array of medications.

Members of the sports emergency care team should be familiar with the EMS professionals who will be responding to a sports emergency and understand the varying levels of care that they provide. In some jurisdictions, EMS is constructed as a 2-tiered system: basic life support (BLS) and advanced life support (ALS). In a 2-tiered system, EMT-Basics respond to all emergency calls, while paramedics units only respond to calls that are determined to need ALS (such as respiratory or cardiac emergencies, unconscious persons). In some jurisdictions, ambulances are staffed with EMT-Paramedics, while others may only utilize EMT-Basics, and EMT-Paramedics respond only when needed. Never assume what the capabilities of the responding EMS squad may be.

PHYSICIANS

Physicians are important members of the sports emergency care team. Athletic trainers work under the supervision of a physician, so close collaboration regarding the implementation between the physician and the athletic trainer is essential. Typically, team physicians are most involved with the development of the sports emergency care team. Team physicians have varying degrees of experience in handling sports emergencies, depending on medical specialty and additional training.

HOSPITAL STAFF

Although it is important to work closely with team physicians to develop the sports emergency care team, other physicians such as emergency room (ER) physicians, should also be considered when developing the emergency plan. Ultimately, the ER physicians and nurses will play a key role in the management of the ill or injured athlete when he or she arrives at the hospital, so it is important to include the ER physician and staff in developing the EAP as well as training exercises.

COACHING STAFF

At the very least, coaches should be trained in first aid and CPR in order to assist an athlete until further help arrives. They can also assist the sports emergency care team in the prevention of athletic injuries by promoting proper techniques and practices to the athletes they coach. However, coaches can also play a greater role as a member of the sports emergency care team, especially in situations when there are fewer human resources (such as in a small high school). Coaches can be included in the emergency plan and trained to assist the athletic trainer in techniques such as CPR, splinting, and management of spine-injured athletes. Since coaches have a personal relationship with their athletes, they may also be valuable in helping to keep the injured athlete calm in an emergency.

ATHLETIC TRAINING STUDENTS

Students in athletic training education programs who are at the scene of an emergency can play an important role in managing an emergency. They should be familiar with emergency supplies and equipment and be ready to retrieve such equipment and assist in its use. Athletic training students should be trained in first aid and professional rescuer CPR.

ATHLETICS STAFF

Other nonmedical staff and support personnel play essential roles in the overall management of emergencies in sports. Athletics staff, site managers, grounds crew members, and others can assist in tasks such as ensuring scene safety, crowd control, and allowing access and guiding EMS to the location of the emergency.

ATHLETES

Athletes should not be excluded when developing the EAP. They can loosely be considered a member of the sports emergency care team by knowing what to do and what not to do when a teammate is injured. Athletes should know never to move an injured athlete because doing so can cause further injury. Athletes should also be taught to report all injuries and not ignore symptoms no matter how insignificant they may seem. In some cases medical emergencies such as concussion or intracranial bleeding often present first with mild symptoms.

OTHER PERSONNEL

EAPs should be specifically tailored for each venue. Therefore, there is no limit to the number or type of personnel who are involved in the management of a sports emergency. While the most common members of the sports emergency care team are listed here, it is by all means not intended to be a complete list (Figure 2-1).

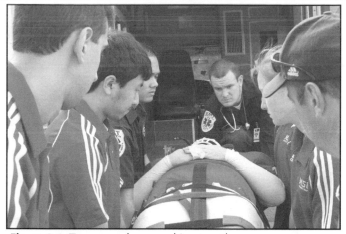

Figure 2-1. Team members working together.

Rules

What rules will be followed when managing an emergency? Is every team member on the same page with regard to protocol? Who is in charge? Will the helmet be removed? These are all questions that must be addressed well in advance of any emergency. The time to argue about protocol for management of an athlete should never take place during an emergency situation. Each member should be included in the development of the EAP to ensure that he or she is comfortable with the protocol that will be used as well as his or her role in the management of an emergency.

Determining how to manage a spine-injured athlete wearing a helmet is of particular importance. While it would appear on paper that athletic trainers, physicians, and EMS personnel are in agreement as to what circumstances warrant helmet removal versus nonremoval, oftentimes local protocols (or even lack of protocols) can be a source of conflict between providers. In 1998, the Inter-Association Task Force for Appropriate Care of the Spine-Injured Athlete published recommendations for management of spinal injuries in athletes wearing protective equipment. The task force consisted of representatives from over 40 professional organizations in the fields of athletic training, emergency medicine, and EMS. These recommendations, which are widely used in sports medicine, agree with the most recent EMT-Basic: National Standard Curriculum. These and other procedural issues must be discussed and agreed upon by members of the team in advance of the start of the season.

Other elements that may seem less critical but are still important include answers to some of the following questions: Who will call 911? Where is the emergency equipment located? Who will retrieve the equipment? Who will

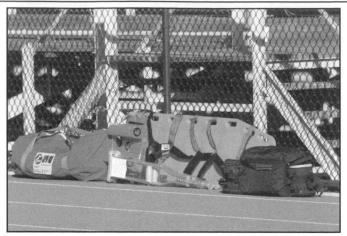

Figure 2-2. Emergency equipment.

guide the ambulance to the scene? Who will notify the athlete's family? Where will the athlete be transported? Of course, this is not a complete list of questions that must be addressed; rather they are suggestions that should prompt the sports emergency care team to think about as many aspects of responding to an emergency as possible in order to develop a comprehensive EAP.

Equipment

Sometimes, the immediate care given to an ill or injured athlete is dependent upon the equipment available at the time of the emergency (Figure 2-2). The sports emergency care team should assess what equipment is needed and what will be available at the venue they are covering. Moreover, all members of the team should be familiar with the location of the equipment, as well as their application and operation. In addition to the usual athletic training supplies, additional emergency equipment that should be considered include the following:

AIRWAY ADJUNCTS

Airway adjuncts include equipment such as a CPR mask, bag-valve mask, oropharyngeal and nasopharyngeal airways, and an advanced airway device (such as a CombiTube [Tyco Healthcare Group, Mansfield, Mass] or a laryngeal mask airway).

BACKBOARDS

Although backboards are standard equipment on an ambulance, the sports emergency care team should consider having a backboard available at venues where there is a higher risk of spinal injury. The team should also take into consideration what size is most suitable, as well as what fastening system (seat belt-style straps versus Velcro [Velcro USA, Inc, Manchester, NH]). Some larger athletes, especially football players wearing protective equipment, may be too large for a standard-sized backboard. Oversize backboards, which are both wider and taller, are available and may be a better choice for larger athletes. One drawback, however, is that oversized backboards may not fit well in some smaller ambulances, and they cannot be used in most medical evacuation helicopters. The sports emergency care team should ensure that equipment that will be used is compatible before the beginning of the season.

SPLINTS

There are several types of commercially available splints, including padded board splints, SAM splints (SAM Medical Products, Newport, Ore), air splints, traction splints, and vacuum splints. Each splinting system has its own advantages and disadvantages. Regardless of the type of splint used, all members of the sports emergency care team should know how to use the splinting system that will be available at the time of an emergency.

COMMUNICATIONS EQUIPMENT

Clear communication is crucial in any emergency situation. In some cases, such as in a high school, athletic trainers may not be able to be present at every activity. In cases such as this, coaches must be able to communicate with athletic trainers if an emergency occurs. While the use of cellular telephones may be suitable in some areas, they may be unreliable in others due to weak cellular signals and should not be relied upon as the only means of communication. The use of portable radios may be a more effective means of communication between coaches and athletic training staff, depending on terrain and area covered. Sports emergency care personnel should know the locations of land line telephones for calling 911. In some cases, EMS systems may consider issuing a portable radio to the athletic training staff for communication in an emergency.

TRANSPORTATION DEVICES

Depending on the severity of the injury or illness, one of a number of different transportation methods may be necessary to move the patient. Crutches, a wheel chair or "sports chair" (a wheel chair designed for use in athletic fields), or a motorized cart may be necessary for minor emergencies. Transportation by ambulance may be necessary in more serious emergencies. Sports emergency care personnel should ensure that these devices or vehicles are available and in working order.

Evacuation via a medical evacuation helicopter may be another option for serious injuries or illnesses that occur in remote locations where transportation times by ground may be excessive or in situations in which the ill or injured athlete requires specialized care that can only be received at a hospital farther away from the scene (such as a trauma or burn center). Sports emergency care personnel should consult with local EMS providers to determine an appropriate area near the venue that can serve as a landing zone.

RESUSCITATION EQUIPMENT

Resuscitation equipment, including an automated external defibrillator (AED) and oxygen, should be available in the event of respiratory or cardiac emergencies. Although ambulances are equipped with AEDs, sports emergency care personnel should ensure that an AED is on hand during athletic events. According to the American Heart Association, chances of survival from cardiac arrest decrease 10% for every minute a shock from a defibrillator is delayed for a victim with a shockable rhythm. If an AED is not available on the field or court, waiting for the ambulance to arrive with an AED can significantly decrease the athlete's chances of survival.

FACEMASK REMOVAL TOOLS

Facemask removal tools should be available at venues where athletes will be wearing helmets with removable facemasks, such as football, lacrosse, and hockey. A universal facemask removal tool such as the FMxtractor (Sports Medicine Concepts, Geneseo, NY) or other tools such as anvil pruners or screwdrivers can aid in facemask removal. Regardless of what facemask removal system is used, sports emergency care personnel must practice frequently with their tool of choice in order to be proficient in its use.

DIAGNOSTIC TOOLS

Assessing an acute injury or illness with diagnostic tools can help provide a more accurate picture of the athlete's condition. Examples of diagnostic tools that should be available include a stethoscope, penlight (to assess pupillary reaction), thermometer, a blood pressure cuff set (including large, regular, and pediatric sizes), and a pulse oximeter.

LIFESAVING MEDICATIONS

In some cases, athletes may carry prescribed lifesaving medications, such as metered dose inhalers, insulin, or Epi-pens (Dey, L.P., Napa, Calif). These medications should be readily accessible on the sideline in the event the athlete needs them. A spare prescription dose and a copy of the prescription should be kept by the athletic trainer if possible and if permitted by local policy.

Planning

Developing the EAP must take all the other PREPARE components into account: what personnel will be involved; what rules will be followed; what equipment will be available; what the arena for the event will be; when the plan will be rehearsed; how will it be evaluated; and what the educational process will be in terms of informing sports emergency care providers, coaches, athletes, and others. The person in charge of developing the EAP should ensure that all stakeholders (eg, administrators, coaches, EMS providers) are part of the planning process. The EAP should be distributed to all members of the sports emergency care team and athletics staff and should also be posted at each venue. Visiting teams should also be provided with a copy of the EAP.

The EAP need not be a lengthy document. However, it should provide detailed instructions as to who will act, what actions will be taken, and how and where they will be taken (Table 2-1). A separate venue-specific EAP should be developed for each venue, complete with detailed instructions and information including but not limited to the address of the venue, a description of the location of emergency equipment, telephone locations, a list of emergency phone numbers, a list of emergency hand signals (for use on the field), and detailed instructions for staff and sports emergency care personnel.

Arena

A separate EAP must be designed for each venue, or "arena," because each arena is unique. Sports emergency care personnel must be familiar with the arena in which the athletic event will occur. Sports emergency care personnel should identify the following prior to any event:

- Condition of the court or field (to identify any potential hazards)
- Location of emergency exits and other routes of egress
- Location of ambulance (if present) or entrance where ambulance or EMS personnel will arrive
- Location of emergency equipment

Consideration must be given as to how an athlete will be transported from the field of play. It may be possible at some outdoor venues for the ambulance to drive on the field. However, sports emergency care personnel must assess the field conditions prior to the game to ensure vehicles will not become stuck if the field is wet. Other venues such as an ice rink may present hazardous conditions for rescuers. Rescuers must prepare for extrication from the field of play in advance and work to minimize any hazards (Figure 2-3).

Rehearsal

An EAP is only useful if it is rehearsed. Frequent practice with all members of the sports medicine team must occur in order for the plan to work

Table 2-1

SAMPLE EMERGENCY ACTION PLAN

_____ University Sports Medicine Football Emergency Protocol

1. Call 911 or other emergency number consistent with organizational policies.
2. Instruct emergency medical services (EMS) personnel to "report to _____ and meet _____ at _____ as we have an injured student-athlete in need of emergency medical treatment."

   University Football Practice Complex: _____ Street entrance (gate across street from _____) cross street: _____ Street

   University Stadium: Gate _____ entrance off _____ Road
3. Provide necessary information to EMS personnel:
   - Name, address, telephone number of caller
   - Number of victims; condition of victims
   - First-aid treatment initiated
   - Specific directions as needed to locate scene
   - Other information as requested by dispatcher
4. Provide appropriate emergency care until arrival of EMS personnel; on arrival of EMS personnel, provide pertinent information (method of injury, vital signs, treatment rendered, medical history) and assist with emergency care as needed.

Note:
   - Sports medicine staff member should accompany student-athlete to hospital
   - Notify other sports medicine staff immediately
   - Parents should be contacted by sports medicine staff
   - Inform coach(es) and administration
   - Obtain medical history and insurance information
   - Appropriate injury reports should be completed

Emergency Telephone Numbers

Hospital	_____ - _____
Emergency Department	_____ - _____
University Health Center	_____ - _____
Campus Police	_____ - _____

Emergency Signals

Physician: arm extended overhead with clenched fist

Paramedics: point to location in end zone by home locker and wave onto field

(continued)

Table 2-1 (continued)
SAMPLE EMERGENCY ACTION PLAN

Spine board: arms held horizontally
Stretcher: supinated hands in front of body or waist level
Splints: hand to lower leg or thigh

Reprinted with permission of National Athletic Trainers' Association.

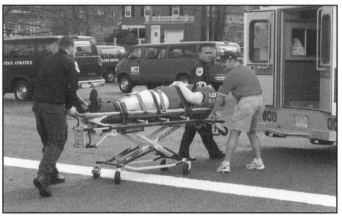

Figure 2-3. The location of the ambulance near the field is important.

effectively (Figure 2-4). The only way to improve response to emergencies and to detect deficiencies in a plan is to identify them through practice. Rehearsing a number of different types of situations will help prepare the team for emergencies. At a minimum, rehearsal should occur before the season begins and should incorporate as many scenarios as possible. Rehearsing scenarios that involve as many members of the sports emergency care team as possible will allow the members of the team to become more comfortable working together and increase the likelihood of a smooth working relationship at the time of an emergency, which ultimately provides for better patient care.

Evaluate and Educate

After rehearsing emergency scenarios, and after every actual emergency, the sports emergency care team should evaluate the event to determine how well the EAP worked, how well the team performed, and what unforeseen factors

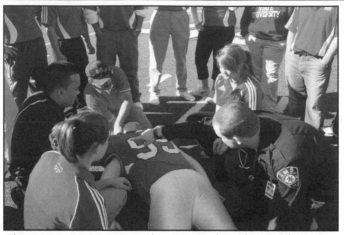

Figure 2-4. Practicing together is crucial in planning for sports emergencies.

affected the incident. An after-action report should be completed by the athletic trainer and shared with all members of the team. In some situations, it may be appropriate to have a debriefing after the incident, so that all members of the team can discuss how the incident was handled and how patient care can be improved in the future. The conclusions from the after-action report, as well as the recommendations from the debriefing, should be considered when updating the EAP.

The EAP should be a living document; it should be evaluated throughout the year and updated whenever necessary. Changes to the venue, changes to telephone numbers, and procedural changes may happen over time. It is critical that the EAP incorporates these changes when they happen.

Bibliography

Anderson JC, Courson RW, Kleiner DM, McLoda TA. National Athletic Trainers' Association position statement: emergency planning in athletics. *Journal of Athletic Training.* 2002;37(1):99-104.

National Highway Traffic Safety Administration. EMT-basic: national standard curriculum. June 2005. Available at: http://www.nhtsa.dot.gov/people/injury/ems/pub/emtbnsc.pdf. Accessed November 2, 2006.

National Highway Traffic Safety Administration. First responder: national standard curriculum. June 2005. Available at: http://www.nhtsa.dot.gov/people/injury/ems/pub/frnsc.pdf. Accessed November 2, 2006.

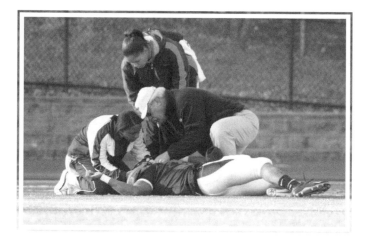

Assessment of Sports Emergencies

Chapter 3

Robb S. Rehberg, PhD, ATC, CSCS, NREMT

Proper assessment of sports injury and illness is an essential skill for health care providers covering sporting events. Rapid assessment on the field can speed appropriate care and mean the difference between life and death in some cases. Immediate assessment of an injury immediately following the traumatic event often reveals clinical indicators that may not be present if proper assessment is delayed due to factors such as swelling, muscle guarding, etc. Moreover, rapid assessment facilitates proper and immediate treatment. A delay in treatment can often complicate an injury (as in a dislocation with muscle spasm) or even decrease chances of survival (as in cardiac arrest).

Various assessment methods will be introduced in this chapter. Many of these assessment tools are designed to uncover signs and symptoms that will be useful in determining the nature of the illness or injury. It is important to note that regardless of the injury or illness, signs and symptoms are like different colors in a detailed painting. The more colors used to paint a picture, the more detailed the painting becomes and the easier it is for the viewer to understand what the painting depicts. The same is true when assessing an ill or injured victim. Usually, one symptom is not enough to determine the condition. It usually takes several signs and symptoms to clearly paint the picture and illustrate the condition.

Mechanism of Injury

In many cases, proper assessment of an athletic injury does not begin when the athletic trainer reaches the athlete. Rather, it begins before athlete contact, at the moment the injury occurs. When covering an athletic event, athletic trainers, EMS personnel, physicians, and other on-field medical staff are in a unique position to actually see the injury occur, a luxury that most health care professionals do not have. We will discuss in this chapter the importance of interviewing the injured athlete about how the injury occurred; however, oftentimes a witnessed mechanism of injury can be just as valuable. In cases in which an athlete is unconscious, a witnessed mechanism of injury by sports medicine personnel can be invaluable in determining the injury.

It is not enough for sports medicine personnel to merely be present at an athletic event. They must have an understanding of the game, know what to look for, and pay close attention to the field of play. Sports medicine personnel should always position themselves where they have an optimum view of the field of play and can view as many athletes as possible. This is especially true in football. Athletic trainers should resist the urge to stand at the line of scrimmage or in a crowd. Instead, the athletic trainer should trail the team he or she is covering to ensure that he or she can visualize every player on the field (Figure 3-1).

Approaching the Athlete: First Steps

Prior to assessing any athlete, the athletic trainer should ensure that he or she has taken proper precautions to protect him- or herself from harm and from disease. Rescuers should approach any injured person with open eyes, paying attention not only to the patient but also to the environment surrounding the patient. Athletic events are usually a controlled environment; however, certain conditions can create a harmful situation for both the injured athlete and the athletic trainer. Athletic trainers should survey the scene and pay particular attention to hazards such as weather conditions, unstable surfaces, and uncontrolled crowds. Always remember that while it is important to provide rapid intervention in an emergency situation, rescuers must always place their own safety first.

It is a given that athletic trainers have disposable examination gloves readily available. However, in situations where there is a reasonable anticipation of exposure to potentially infectious material such as blood or body fluids containing blood, athletic trainers may require additional personal protective equipment. In addition to gloves, items such as face shields, gowns, and masks may be necessary (Figure 3-2). Athletic trainers should always minimize their exposure to blood or other potentially infectious materials by following the Occupational Safety and Health Administration's Bloodborne Pathogens Standard (29 CFR 1910.1030). Likewise, athletic trainers must be aware of the potential risk of airborne pathogens and take precautions to minimize exposure. This is especially true when assessing or treating an injury around the mouth and nose (Figure 3-3).

Try to determine the mechanism of injury as you approach the victim. If you did not witness the mechanism of injury, you may need to rely on

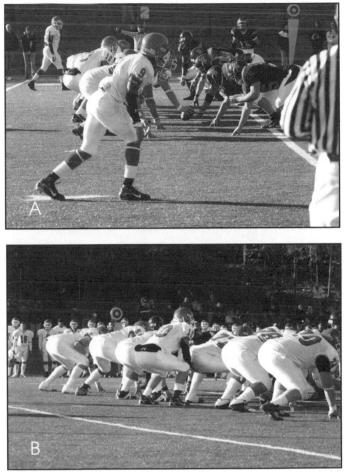

Figure 3-1. Trailing the action provides a better view of the field of play.

bystanders and the victim's recollection of the event. If the victim is suffering from an illness, try to determine the nature of the illness.

Initial Assessment

Regardless of the mechanism of injury, the athletic trainer should always assess immediate life threats first. Immediate life threats are symptoms that must be addressed immediately to sustain life. Assessing for immediate life threats begins with checking the athlete's mental status. A victim's mental status is determined by using the AVPU scale (Table 3-1).

Figure 3-2. Personal protective equipment.

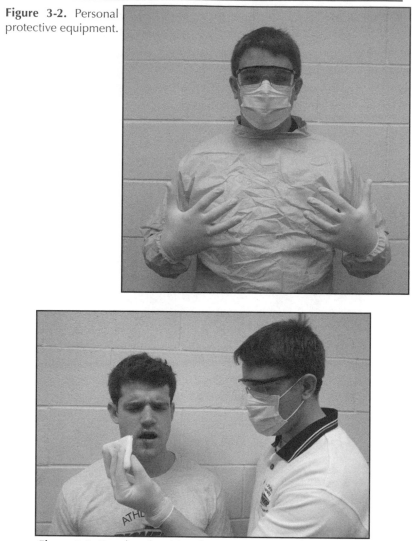

Figure 3-3. Stand to the side when treating a mouth injury.

Table 3-1

ASSESSING LEVEL OF CONSCIOUSNESS: THE AVPU SCALE

* Alert: victim is alert and oriented
* Verbal: victim responds to verbal stimuli
* Painful: victim responds to painful stimuli
* Unresponsive

- A—Alert: If a victim is alert, assess whether he or she is oriented to time (what time is it?), place (where is he or she?), person (who is he or she?), and event (what is he or she doing?). This is often documented as being conscious, alert, and oriented times four (often documented as CAOx4). The inability of a victim to recognize time, place, person, and/or event may be an indication of a brain injury.

- V—Verbal: The victim responds to verbal stimuli only. This means that the victim is unresponsive, but responds when the rescuer speaks to him or her. In this case, the victim may appear to be unconscious but does respond to questions when asked by the rescuer.

- P—Painful: The victim is unresponsive and does not respond to questions asked by the rescuer but does respond when a painful stimulus is applied. An example of a painful stimulus might be rubbing the sternum or pinching the nail bed of the victim's thumb.

- U—Unresponsive: The victim is unconscious and unresponsive to verbal or painful stimuli.

Once the victim's mental status is determined, the athletic trainer should continue the initial assessment by checking for and correcting immediate life threats. All health care providers are familiar with the initial assessment of airway, breathing, and circulation (ABC), and some health care providers follow an assessment algorithm that adds deformity (D) and exposure (E). Because of the unique nature of the types of emergencies common to sports, a variation of the ABC algorithm is recommended. The ABC Sx3 (ABC, S times three) algorithm (Table 3-2) adds 3 important components to the initial assessment: checking for and treating severe bleeding, shock, and spinal injury. Using the ABC Sx3 algorithm allows the athletic trainer to quickly identify and treat immediate life threats in order of severity.

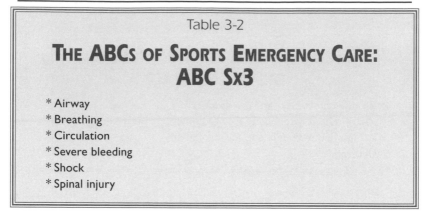

Table 3-2

THE ABCs OF SPORTS EMERGENCY CARE: ABC Sx3

* Airway
* Breathing
* Circulation
* Severe bleeding
* Shock
* Spinal injury

AIRWAY

If the patient is found to be alert, the athletic trainer knows that the athlete has an airway, is breathing, and has a pulse. A quick scan of the body for severe bleeding, a visual inspection of the skin temperature and condition, assessing capillary refill, and a cursory motor/sensory assessment can also rule out other immediate life threats. However, if a victim is unresponsive, the athletic trainer must ensure the victim has a patent airway. Open the airway by using either a head-tilt chin-lift or a jaw thrust if a spinal injury is suspected (Figure 3-4). Rescuers may consider using airway adjuncts to keep the airway open. This will be discussed further in Chapter 4. The airway must be protected at all times regardless of the nature of the injury or illness.

BREATHING

Once the airway is open, rescuers should assess for breathing. If breathing is absent, rescue breathing should be performed as per the most current guidelines for CPR and emergency cardiovascular care. If the victim is breathing, the athletic trainer should note the rate and quality of breathing. Breathing rates of less than 8 and greater than 30 require ventilatory support. This will be discussed further in Chapter 4.

CIRCULATION

Assess the victim's pulse at the carotid artery. If there is no pulse, begin CPR and if equipped, use an AED as per the most recent guidelines for CPR and emergency cardiovascular care. If a pulse is present, note the rate and quality of the pulse (ie, rapid and weak, slow and strong). There is some evidence in

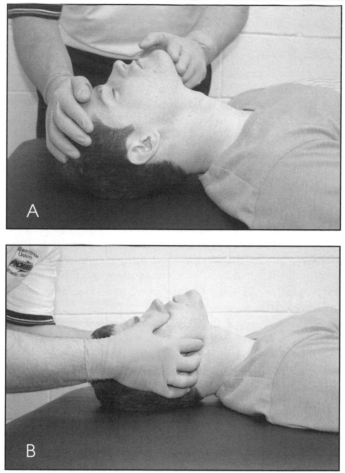

Figure 3-4. (A) Head-tilt chin-lift. (B) Modified jaw thrust.

the literature that suggests the presence of a palpable pulse at the carotid artery is an indication of a systolic blood pressure of at least 80 mm Hg.[1]

SEVERE BLEEDING

Quickly assess for severe bleeding, and control bleeding by using direct pressure. Quickly limiting severe blood loss can increase the patient's chances of survival. When assessing for severe bleeding, it is important to assess the entire body.

SHOCK

In addition to assessing pulse and breathing rate and quality, there are several key signs of shock that rescuers should assess, including skin color, skin temperature and condition, and capillary refill. These quick assessments will help the rescuer form a general impression of how adequately the victim is perfusing oxygenated blood throughout the body. Changes in normal skin complexion, such as pale, cyanotic, flushed, red, or jaundice skin, may be an indication of shock. Skin temperature and moisture (eg, hot and dry or cool and clammy) may also be indicators of shock.

SPINAL INJURY

A cursory assessment of motor and sensory function in the extremities should be performed next. While a more detailed neurological examination will be discussed later, a brief assessment of sensory and motor function in the extremities, combined with the mechanism of injury and the victim's chief complaint, will help determine whether or not spinal precautions will be necessary. A spinal injury should be suspected in all traumatic injuries until proven otherwise.

Assess for sensory nerve function by brushing or gently pinching the victim's hands and feet. The athletic trainer should ask the victim to squeeze his or her fingers with his or her hands and plantar flex his or her ankle against resistance to assess motor function. The absence of sensory and/or motor function does not conclusively indicate a spinal injury. Nonetheless, spinal precautions must be taken in any situation where a sensory or motor deficit is present. Conversely, although a victim's ability to feel sensation and provide resistance indicates that spinal injury is not likely, it does not rule out a spinal fracture that may endanger the spinal cord if managed poorly. The sports emergency care team must complete a thorough assessment and take appropriate precautions based on their findings. Additional information on management of spinal injuries is found in Chapter 6.

Focused History and Physical Examination/Rapid Assessment

Once immediate life threats are assessed, the sports emergency care team member should focus on the injury or illness. If the injury or illness is obvious, the athletic trainer can perform a focused history and physical examination by obtaining a SAMPLE history (Signs/Symptoms, Allergies, Medications, Past medical history, Last oral intake, Events leading to the injury/illness) (Table 3-3), examining the injured area (including performing any necessary special tests), and obtaining a set of baseline vital signs (including but not

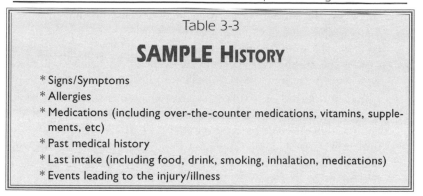

Table 3-3

SAMPLE History

* Signs/Symptoms
* Allergies
* Medications (including over-the-counter medications, vitamins, supplements, etc)
* Past medical history
* Last intake (including food, drink, smoking, inhalation, medications)
* Events leading to the injury/illness

limited to pulse, respiratory rate, and blood pressure). Since most traumatic injuries in sports are not multiple systems trauma in nature (meaning several body systems are involved), it is usually easy to quickly identify the injured area and move directly to focused history and physical examination. However, there may be situations in which more than one body system is injured or the victim is unable to verbalize the location of the injury. In these situations, a rapid trauma assessment consisting of a head-to-toe examination and baseline vital signs should be performed. The athletic trainer should keep in mind that this algorithm for assessment is designed for emergencies. Other serious but nonemergent conditions (such as a shoulder dislocation or an anterior cruciate ligament [ACL] sprain) may not require a comprehensive assessment as described here.

SAMPLE History

If the injury or illness is obvious, begin the focused history and assessment by asking the athlete about his or her chief complaint (what hurts) and beginning an examination of the injured area and a SAMPLE history. The SAMPLE acronym can help rescuers systematically obtain necessary medical information in an emergency situation. Prehospital care providers have used the SAMPLE history for several years. Athletic trainers who obtain a SAMPLE history and are able to convey these findings during the transfer of care will present the necessary information in a format that is familiar to EMS personnel. It is important to be thorough when obtaining a medical history and to ask the right questions in order to receive the complete picture. For instance, it is not enough to ask a victim, "Do you take any medications?" While that question may prompt some victims to provide a very thorough answer, others may not consider over-the-counter medications and supplements worth mentioning. Rescuers should choose their words carefully and pay close attention to the victim's responses when obtaining a medical history from a victim.

Taking a SAMPLE history includes the following information:

- Signs/symptoms: Signs (something the rescuer can see) will be uncovered by performing a quick visual inspection. Further assessment of signs will occur during the detailed assessment. The patient will reveal symptoms (something the victim tells you) during the interview.

- Allergies: Ask the victim if he or she has any known allergies. Allergies to penicillin-based or sulfa-based medications will be significant to note because this may be a cause of the illness. This information may also impact the patient's care so as not to administer medication to which the patient may be allergic. Food allergies such as to shellfish or nuts may be relevant to uncovering the nature of the illness. Seasonal allergies should also be noted because they could also be a contributing factor. Allergies to fabrics and other synthetic materials should also be noted. (Rubber is a material to be aware of with the prevalence of synthetic turf fields, many of which contain rubber.) Awareness of latex allergies is important as well. Sports emergency care providers should be sure to have nonlatex examination gloves readily available.

- Medications: Ask the victim what medications he or she is taking, including prescription and over-the-counter medications, vitamins, supplements, and herbal remedies. Note the last time the victim ingested a medication as well as the amount taken. This information is important for several reasons because the victim may require additional medication or surgery, the victim may be directed to take a medication but has missed one or more doses, or the medication may be a contributing factor to the present illness.

- Past medical history: Any significant past medical history, including major or chronic illnesses, surgeries, or hospitalization, should be noted. While obtaining a thorough history is of value to the medical staff at the receiving hospital, past medical history may provide important clues as to the nature of the present illness.

- Last intake: When was the last time the patient ate, drank, smoked, chewed tobacco, or placed any substance in his or her mouth? Note the time and quantity of each. Once again, this information may provide clues as to the history of the present illness. It will also be valuable to the receiving medical staff in the event surgery is necessary.

- Events leading to the injury/illness: Asking the victim if he or she remembers the events leading to the injury or illness can prove valuable in determining the cause. While information from bystanders regarding the incident can also be valuable, it is important to determine whether the victim can remember the events by him- or herself. After the victim provides information, ask him or her, "Is that what you remember happening, or is that what others told you?" The inability to remember the events leading to the injury or illness may be a significant clinical indicator. Moreover, a thorough history must include questions regarding the event in order to ascertain the exact cause. For instance, if you find a victim with a head injury having seizures, did the victim have a seizure and subsequently hit his or her head or did an injury to the head cause the seizure?

Obtaining Additional Information: OPQRST

In some situations, obtaining information on the characteristics of the pain experienced by the injured athlete may assist the athletic trainer during the assessment process. OPQRST (Onset, Provocation/Palliation, Quality, Region/Radiation, Severity, Time) is another commonly used acronym by prehospital care providers that is useful in assessing pain characteristics.

- Onset: What time did the pain begin? Did the pain begin suddenly, or did it come gradually?
- Provocation/palliation: What was the victim doing when the pain began? Did the victim do something to cause the pain? Is there anything that makes the pain worse? Is there anything that relieves the pain?
- Quality: What does the pain feel like? Oftentimes, pain is characterized as sharp, dull, aching, throbbing, stabbing, shooting, or intermittent. Understanding the type of pain may hold clues to the condition producing the pain.
- Region/radiation: Where is the pain? Where does the pain begin? Is it localized or diffuse? Does it radiate to another part of the body?
- Severity: How severe is the pain? How does it compare to previous injuries? Often, a scale of 1 to 10 is used to assess pain. (While this scale is useful to determine whether pain increases or decreases, it is subjective in nature and thus not reliable as an indicator to the type of injury/illness.)
- Time: When did the pain begin? How long does the pain last?

Rapid Trauma Assessment

If the injury or illness is not immediately known, a rapid trauma assessment should be performed. Beginning at the head and working toward the toes, the athletic trainer should visually inspect and palpate for abnormalities (Table 3-4). During the assessment, the athletic trainer should look for DCAP-BTLS: Deformities, Contusions, Abrasions, Punctures/Penetrations, Burns, Tenderness, Lacerations, and Swelling.[2] Assessment for other body-area specific conditions should also be performed.

Table 3-4

HEAD-TO-TOE ASSESSMENT

Body Area	Assess For
Head	DCAP-BTLS plus pupillary response, drainage or bleeding from ears or nose, and crepitation
Eyes	DCAP-BTLS plus foreign bodies and blood in anterior chamber (hyphema)
Mouth	DCAP-BTLS plus dislodged teeth, airway obstructions, swollen or lacerated tongue, odors, and discoloration
Neck	DCAP-BTLS plus jugular vein distension (JVD) and crepitation
Chest	DCAP-BTLS plus paradoxical motion, crepitation, and breath sounds (presence, absence, equality)
Abdomen	DCAP-BTLS plus note firmness, softness, and distension
Pelvis	DCAP-BTLS plus check for pelvic stability
Extremities	DCAP-BTLS plus assess distal pulse, sensation, motor function, and medic alert tags

Obtaining Vital Signs

Vital signs such as pulse, respirations, and blood pressure can be key in determining how efficiently the body is functioning. Vital signs that fall outside normal range limits may be an indication of severe or acute injury or illness. A set of baseline vital signs, including but not limited to pulse, respirations, and blood pressure, should be taken. Continuous reassessment of vital signs should be performed throughout treatment and transportation to the hospital. Table 3-5 lists the normal range limits for vital signs in healthy individuals. However, the athletic trainer should be reminded that normal resting vital signs in elite athletes might be lower than that of the average person. Conversely, athletes who were actively participating in their sport just prior to assessment may present with vital signs that are higher than the normal limits.

PULSE

While the presence of a pulse was assessed during the initial assessment by palpating the carotid artery, assessing for a pulse at the radial artery is a useful diagnostic tool (Figure 3-5A). As mentioned earlier, presence of a radial pulse represents a systolic blood pressure of at least 80 mm Hg. Note the rate and quality of the pulse felt when assessing a radial pulse. The rate should be

Table 3-5

NORMAL VITAL SIGN VALUES
IN HEALTHY INDIVIDUALS

	Adult	*Adolescent (11 years to 14 years)*	*Child (6 years to 10 years)*
Pulse (per minute)	60 to 100	60 to 105	70 to 110
Respirations (per minute)	12 to 20	12 to 20	15 to 30
Systolic blood pressure (mm Hg)	90 to 140	88 to 140	80 to 122
Diastolic blood pressure (mm Hg)	60 to 90	Approximately 2/3 of systolic pressure in adolescents and children	
Temperature	~ 98.6°F for all ages		
Capillary refill	<3 seconds for all ages		
Pulse oximetry (for all ages)	95% to 100% Normal		
	91% to 94% Mild hypoxia		
	86% to 90% Moderate hypoxia		
	<85% Severe hypoxia		

Vital Sign Changes With Exercise

Vital Sign	Exercising Person
Pulse	Faster and stronger
Respirations	Faster and deeper
Blood pressure (systolic)	Elevated
Blood pressure (diastolic)	About the same
Skin color	Flushed if warm and sweating, grey or whitish if cold
Skin temperature	Cool with sweat or hypothermia, warm to hot if flushed or heat stroke
Sweating	Present, could be significant

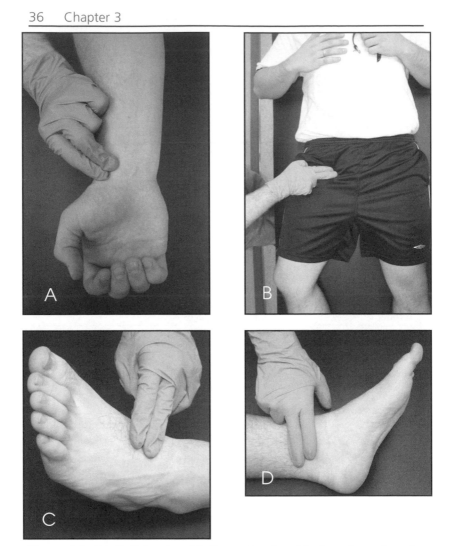

Figure 3-5. (A) Radial pulse. (B) Femoral pulse. (C) Dorsalis pedis pulse. (D) Anterior tibial pulse.

determined by counting the number of beats for 30 seconds and multiplying by 2 to determine the number of beats per minute. Also note the strength of the pulse. Is the pulse bounding (strong) or thready (weak)? If a radial pulse cannot be felt, assess for a pulse at the femoral artery (Figure 3-5B). For severe injuries to the lower extremity, presence of a pulse at the dorsalis pedis (Figure 3-5C) or anterior tibial location (Figure 3-5D) may be necessary.

RESPIRATIONS

Assess respirations by watching the athlete's chest rise and fall. In some instances, it may be helpful to place a hand on the athlete's chest to aid in assessing respirations. Assess breathing for 30 seconds and multiply by 2 to determine breaths per minute. While assessing respirations, note whether or not the chest expands symmetrically on both sides. Also note the quality of breaths (eg, normal versus labored, deep versus shallow, regular versus irregular). Assessment of lung sounds via auscultation will be discussed in Chapter 4.

BLOOD PRESSURE

Blood pressure is the key diagnostic test that determines a victim's condition in an emergency. Assessment of blood pressure can be performed using 2 different methods: auscultation (preferred) or palpation. Assessing blood pressure by auscultation is preferred because it provides a more accurate reading, and both the systolic and diastolic values can be obtained. Assessing blood pressure by palpation only produces a systolic value and may be less accurate. While auscultation is the preferred method of blood pressure assessment, assessing blood pressure by palpation does offer advantages in situations where noise from a crowded stadium or arena may prevent an accurate auscultative reading. Although assessment by palpation does not produce a diastolic value, it is the systolic value that is of greater importance in emergency situations.

It is important that the correct cuff size is used when performing a blood pressure assessment. Standard size blood cuffs should not be used in patients with an upper arm circumference of more than 34 cm.[3] Sports emergency care providers should be prepared for any size athlete and should have access to different cuff sizes, including pediatric, regular, and large cuffs.

Blood Pressure by Auscultation

Place the sphygmomanometer cuff around the upper arm and just above the elbow. Follow the directions on the cuff for proper placement, if present. Secure the cuff snugly around the arm. Place the earpieces of the stethoscope in your ears and place the bell of the stethoscope over the brachial artery at the medial aspect of the antecubital space (Figure 3-6A). Next, close the valve and inflate the cuff. As the cuff inflates, a pulse will be audible. Continue to inflate the cuff until the audible pulse disappears, then continue to inflate the cuff at least 30 mm Hg further. Slowly release air from the valve at a rate of about 5 mm Hg to 10 mm Hg per second. Note the reading at which the first audible pulse is heard. This is the systolic value. Continue to steadily release air from the bladder until the audible pulse disappears and note the reading when it does. This is the diastolic value.

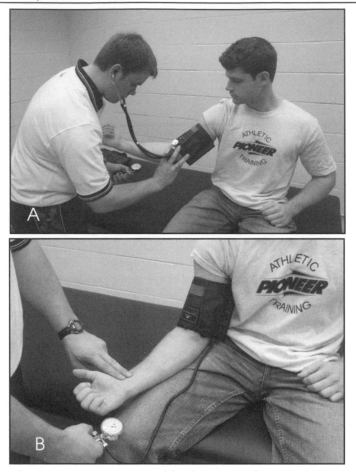

Figure 3-6. (A) Assessing blood pressure by auscultation. (B) Assessing blood pressure by palpation.

Blood Pressure by Palpation

Place the sphygmomanometer in the same manner described above. Next, palpate the radial pulse (Figure 3-6B). Once the radial pulse is felt, inflate the cuff until you can no longer feel the radial pulse. Then, inflate the cuff an additional 30 mm Hg to 40 mm Hg past that point. Finally, while still keeping your fingers in place to palpate the radial pulse, slowly begin releasing air from the cuff at a rate of about 5 mm Hg to 10 mm Hg per second. Note the pressure at which the radial pulse returns. This is the systolic value. For instance, if the pulse returns at 140 mm Hg, the blood pressure is 140 by palpation, or 140/p.

Other Significant Diagnostic Signs

There are other diagnostic signs that are useful in determining the athlete's overall condition (see Table 3-5).

SKIN ASSESSMENT

Assessing the skin for color (pallor), temperature, and moisture can be of particular importance. Pale skin (or loss of normal skin complexion in darker skinned individuals) may be an indication of shock. Flushed, red skin may be an indication of heat illness, anaphylaxis, hypertension, or emotional distress. Clammy or moist skin may indicate shock as well. Hot skin may indicate heat illness or fever, cool skin may indicate shock, and cold skin may indicate prolonged cold exposure.

PULSE OXIMETRY

Use of a pulse oximeter is helpful in determining how adequately oxygen is perfusing throughout the body. The pulse oximeter is a device that measures oxygen saturation using a photoelectric sensor that attaches to the athlete's finger or ear. There are several types of pulse oximeters available that range in price and size. Sports emergency care providers should consider having a pulse oximeter as standard equipment.

CAPILLARY REFILL

If a pulse oximeter is not present, the capillary refill test can be used as a method to assess perfusion of oxygenated blood to the extremities. When a victim is in shock, the body shunts blood away from the skin. The capillary refill test, also known as the blanch test, is performed by pressing on the nail bed until it turns white (Figure 3-7A). This forces oxygenated blood out of the tissues being depressed. In victims with adequate perfusion, blood should return to the underlying tissue and the nail bed should return to its normal pink color within 2 seconds (Figure 3-7B). A capillary refill time greater than 2 seconds is a sign of inadequate perfusion and may be an indication of shock, dehydration, hypothermia, or a peripheral vascular disease.

TEMPERATURE

Temperature should be assessed whenever fever or environmental emergencies such as heat illness or hypothermia are suspected. In the field, temperature should be assessed orally or with the use of a tympanic thermometer. If using a tympanic thermometer, the rescuer should be properly trained and proficient in its use. While there are conflicting studies regarding the reliability of

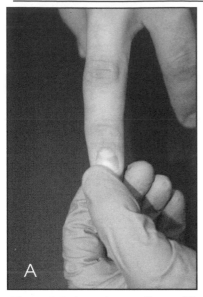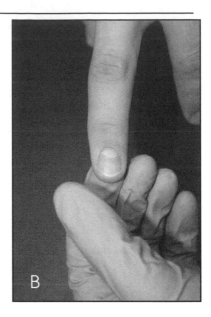

Figure 3-7. Assessing capillary refill.

tympanic thermometers, improper use of tympanic thermometers will contribute to faulty readings. Serial temperature measurements should be obtained in order to ensure an accurate reading.

Vital Sign Trending: The Rule of 100

As stated earlier, signs and symptoms aid in painting a picture of the victim's condition. Each vital sign can be likened to a color in a detailed painting. The more colors used in the painting, the more detail is seen and the picture becomes clearer. The same is true for vital signs. The "Rule of 100" pays particular attention to 3 vital signs in predicting the severity of injury or illness. Specifically, the assessment of pulse, systolic blood pressure, and temperature can be useful in determining serious cardiopulmonary conditions. The "Rule of 100" states that if the systolic blood pressure is greater than 100 and the pulse and temperature are less than 100, significant injury is unlikely. Conversely, a systolic blood pressure of less than 100 and/or a pulse and temperature greater than 100 may indicate a serious injury or illness requiring further medical evaluation. A series of vital sign assessments at intervals of 10 min or less and over at least a 30-min period should be obtained in order to determine trends in the readings obtained.[4]

References

1. American College of Surgeons. *Advanced Trauma Life Support for Doctors*. 6th ed. Chicago, Ill: Author; 1997.
2. National Highway Traffic Safety Administration. Emergency medical technician-basic: national standard curriculum. Available at: http://www.nhtsa.dot.gov/people/injury/ems/pub/emtbnsc.pdf. Accessed March 28, 2007.
3. American Academy of Family Physicians. Medical care for obese patients: advice for health care professionals. *Am Fam Physician.* 2002;65(1):81-88.
4. Kyle J, Leaman J, Courson R, Rehberg R, McGrady T. Sports trauma "red bag" vital sign trending. Available at: http://www.healthgiant.com/shop/ht_sprt-trauma.asp. Accessed July 12, 2006.

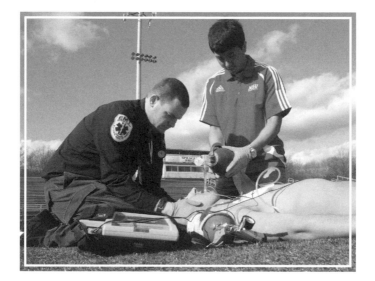

Chapter **4**

Airway Management and Breathing

Robb S. Rehberg, PhD, ATC, CSCS, NREMT

Establishing and maintaining a patent airway are perhaps the most important tasks with which sports emergency care providers are faced. Breathing cannot occur without an airway, and if breathing ceases, so does circulation, and death is the result. There are a multitude of injuries and illnesses that can contribute to respiratory compromise and difficulty breathing, many of which will be covered throughout this book. The sports emergency care team must anticipate that trauma related to sports participation may result in airway and breathing compromise and must have appropriate plans in place to manage such emergencies. This chapter will address methods of establishing and maintaining an airway, as well as the management of respiratory emergencies.

All sports emergency care personnel should be trained and current in professional rescuer basic life support. Professional-level basic life support courses cover content including adult, infant, and child rescue breathing and CPR; foreign body airway obstruction; 2-rescuer resuscitation; and use of adjunctive equipment such as a CPR mask and bag-valve mask. While airway management and breathing are covered in this chapter, it is not intended to be a substitute for skills covered in a professional-level CPR course.

Review of Clinically Relevant Anatomy

In order to successfully manage a patient's airway, sports emergency care providers must have an understanding of the anatomical features of the upper and lower airway (Figure 4-1). Air enters the upper airway via the nose or mouth. The palate separates both airway openings. Behind the nose and above the palate is the nasal floor, which gives rise to the nasopharynx. In the mouth

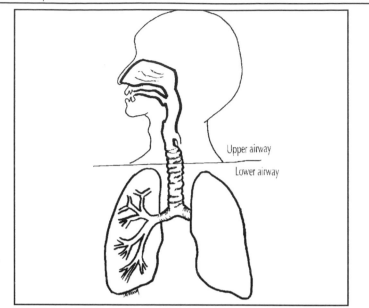

Figure 4-1. Upper and lower airways. (Illustration by Joelle Rehberg, DO.)

(below the palate), the oropharynx runs posteriorly, and both the nasopharynx and the oropharynx join at the posterior aspect of the airway, called the pharynx. The pharynx descends behind the tongue where the epiglottis separates the pharynx and the larynx. The larynx extends past the lower pharynx to the trachea.

The lower airway consists of the right and left main bronchi. Each of the main bronchi branch off to each of the lobes of the lungs (2 on the left and 3 on the right). In the lungs, the bronchi branch off into smaller bronchioles, and finally to alveolar ducts, which are lined with alveoli. The alveoli are small air sacs where gas exchange occurs.

Establishing an Airway

Assessing and establishing a patent airway is the first priority in any emergency. Most conscious victims are able to maintain a patent airway without assistance. If an athlete is able to verbalize any response, we know the airway is open. However, unconscious victims and victims with an altered mental status may need assistance in keeping the airway open. The procedures for airway evaluation (ie, opening the airway and artificial ventilation) should be performed with the patient lying

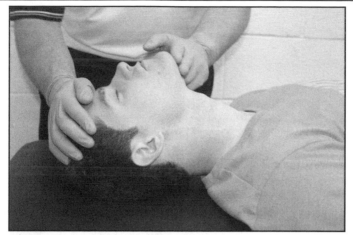

Figure 4-2. Head-tilt chin-lift.

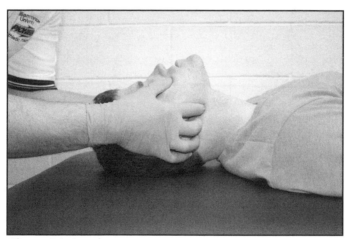

Figure 4-3. Jaw thrust.

supine. The primary method of establishing an open airway is the head-tilt chin-lift. The head-tilt chin-lift is accomplished by placing one hand on the forehead, grasping the bony aspect of the chin with the other hand, and tilting the head and lifting the chin simultaneously (Figure 4-2). The rescuer should be sure to tilt the head so that the jaw is near perpendicular to the ground.

If a spinal injury is suspected, the rescuer should instead use the jaw thrust maneuver. To perform the jaw thrust, place the thumbs on the cheeks and the index and middle fingers behind the angle of the jaw and slide the jaw forward like a drawer (Figure 4-3).

Figure 4-4. (A) Oropharyngeal airway insertion.

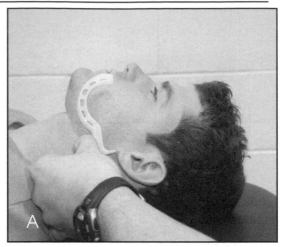

USE OF AIRWAY ADJUNCTS

In some cases, it is difficult to maintain an open airway by using manual methods alone. If a victim requires ventilation, the use of airway adjuncts or advanced airway devices can aid in ensuring a patent airway during resuscitation.

Oropharyngeal airways are effective in maintaining a patent airway in victims who are unconscious and do not have a gag reflex. Oropharyngeal airways should not be used in patents who are conscious or who have a gag reflex because they may cause the victim to vomit. Oropharyngeal airways come in assorted sizes, and the correct size is selected by measuring the distance between the tip of the ear and the corner of the mouth (Figure 4-4A). Once the correct size is selected, the following steps should be followed:

- Place the patient in the supine position with the head in a neutral position.
- Perform a crossed-finger technique. Cross the thumb and forefinger of one hand and place them on the upper and lower teeth at the corner of the athlete's mouth. Spread your fingers apart to open the athlete's mouth.
- Position the airway so that its tip is pointing toward the roof of the patient's mouth.
- Insert the airway and slide it along the roof of the mouth, past the soft tissue hanging down the back, or until you meet resistance against the back of the soft palate.

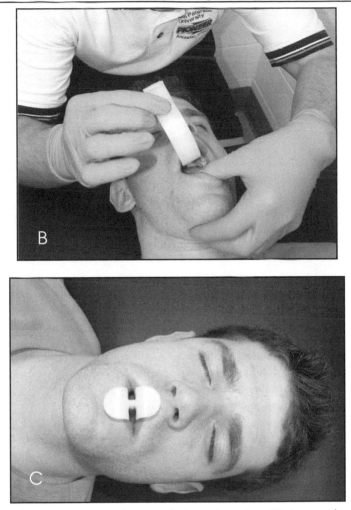

Figure 4-4. (B) Oropharyngeal airway insertion. (C) A properly inserted oropharyngeal airway.

- Gently rotate the airway 180 degrees so that the tip is pointing down into the patient's pharynx (Figure 4-4B).
- Once properly inserted, the end of the oropharyngeal airway will rest just above the lips (Figure 4-4C).

A nasopharyngeal airway is another mechanical airway device that can be used for maintaining a patent airway. Unlike oropharyngeal airways, nasopharyngeal airways are usually better tolerated because they are less likely to produce a gag reflex. Nasopharyngeal airways are measured by selecting an

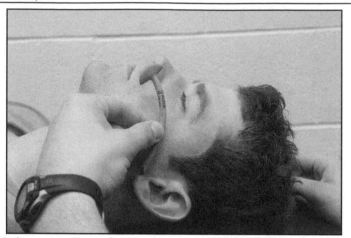

Figure 4-5. Measuring a nasopharyngeal airway.

airway with a diameter similar to that of the nasal passage. This can usually be measured by comparing the airway diameter to that of the patient's fifth finger. Measure the length by measuring from the athlete's nostril to the earlobe or to the angle of the jaw (Figure 4-5). Choosing the correct length also helps ensure the appropriate diameter. Once the correct size has been selected, the following steps should be followed:

- Lubricate the airway with a water-soluble lubricant.
- Keep the patient's head in a neutral position.
- Gently push the tip of the nose upward.
- Insert the airway into the nostril (use the right nostril when possible) with the bevel of the airway toward the septum.

Nasopharyngeal airways should not be used on patients with severe head trauma or where a basal skull fracture may be present.

Advanced airway devices such as a laryngeal mask airway (LMA), Combi-Tube (Figure 4-6), or an endotracheal (ET) tube are a more reliable means of airway management than oropharyngeal and nasopharyngeal airways and are often used by prehospital care personnel in the field. The use of these devices may be restricted depending on state or local regulations. Sports emergency care providers should follow local protocol before considering the use of advanced airway devices for sports emergencies. The LMA and CombiTube are designed for blind insertion unlike an ET tube, which requires the use of a laryngoscope for proper placement. In the prehospital setting, ET tubes are typically inserted by advanced life support personnel such as paramedics. However, depending on local or state regulations, basic life support personnel (and possibly athletic trainers) may be permitted to insert an LMA or

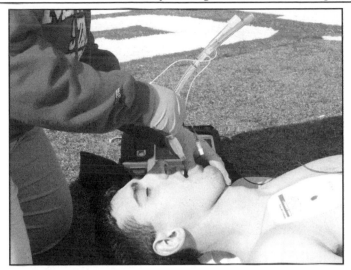

Figure 4-6. CombiTube.

CombiTube if trained. Be sure to check local protocol and existing regulations before considering the use of an advanced airway.

Sports emergency care personnel should be prepared to clear the airway in the event the patient vomits. Aspiration of vomitus into the airway is a serious complication that can hamper resuscitation efforts and cause further injury to the patient. In the event a patient vomits, suction may be necessary to clear the airway. Suction devices should be readily available for use. There are 3 different types of suction units that are typically used in the prehospital setting. Battery-powered suction units are often carried by EMS units and operate using a pump that is powered by a rechargeable battery (Figure 4-7A). Oxygen-powered suction units create suction from the flow of oxygen and do not rely on batteries or electricity for power. Manual suction units (Figure 4-7B) are compact and inexpensive and can easily be kept in a medical kit.

There are different types of suction catheters that can be used for suctioning. The most common types are flexible (also known as French) or rigid (also known as Yankauer).

Indications for suctioning include vomiting in an unresponsive patient, in a patient with an altered mental status, or in a patient who has been secured to a spine board. Before suctioning begins, the maximum depth that the suction catheter is to be inserted should be measured using the distance from the corner of the mouth to the earlobe. The suction catheter should not be inserted deeper than this measurement. Suctioning should then be performed by inserting the catheter and using a figure eight motion. For powered suction

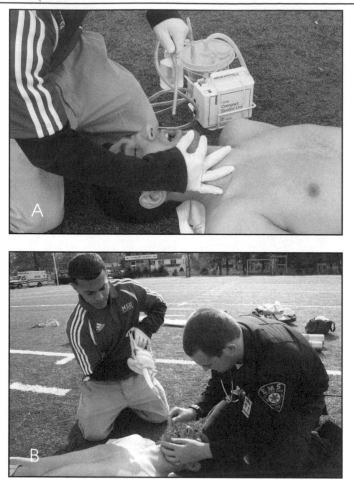

Figure 4-7. (A) Battery-powered suction unit. (B) Manual suction unit.

units, inserting the catheter in sterile water before and after suctioning is recommended in order to clean the catheter and decrease the chances of blockage. Do not suction for more than 10 seconds at a time.

Assessing Breathing

When assessing for the presence of breathing, rescuers look for chest rise and listen and feel for breathing. However, once the primary assessment has been completed and airway, breathing, and circulation are confirmed, a more

Table 4-1	
RESTING RESPIRATORY RATES (PER MINUTE)	
Adult	12 to 20
Adolescent	12 to 20
Child <10 years old	15 to 30

detailed assessment of breathing will be necessary. Specifically, assessment of breathing rate and quality is usually performed during a detailed physical examination. Table 4-1 lists normal respiratory rates by age; however, it is important to realize that athletes who have been participating in physical activity may present with higher respiratory rates. The respiratory rate can be assessed by counting the number of times the chest rises and falls in a 30-second period and multiplying it by 2. Additionally, sports emergency care personnel may choose to use a stethoscope to determine respiratory rate.

In addition to respiratory rate, respiratory quality should be assessed by observing the patient and by listening to breath sounds. Patients in respiratory distress may exhibit visual signs such as nasal flaring, intercostal retractions, and cyanosis. Sports emergency care personnel should assess breath sounds over both the anterior and posterior aspects of the chest (Figure 4-8). Breath sounds in a healthy person should be clear and equal over both lungs. Breath sounds should always be assessed before and after insertion of an advanced airway to ensure proper placement.

Absent, diminished, or abnormal breath sounds may indicate respiratory compromise. Common abnormal breath sounds that may be present include rales, rhonchi, and wheezing. Rales, a wet crackling noise, are a sign of fluid in the lungs. Rales are often heard in patients with pneumonia. Rhonchi are coarse rattling or snoring sounds, indicative of inflammation or secretions in the bronchial tubes. Wheezing is a high-pitched, musical sound that is an indication of narrowed airway passages. Wheezing is typically heard during inhalation and exhalation.

While the presence of abnormal breath sounds alone may not be sufficient to form a clinical impression, they do serve as valuable clues when combined with other symptoms. Sports emergency care personnel should note respiratory rate and quality, and reassess every 5 minutes.

Breathing Support

The primary assessment begins with assessing airway, breathing, and circulation. If breathing is absent, or if breathing and pulse are both absent, rescue breathing or CPR will be required. Rescue breathing or CPR should be

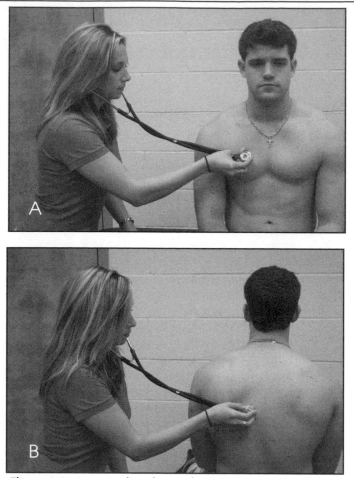

Figure 4-8. Assessing breath sounds.

administered per the most recent CPR guidelines and should be delivered using either a CPR mask (Figure 4-9) or a bag-valve mask (Figure 4-10).

If breathing is present, the rate, quality, and equality of breathing should be assessed. Patients whose respiratory rate is less than 8 breaths per minute may need supplemental ventilation. Patients whose respiratory rate is greater than 20 breaths per minute may need assistance in regaining control of breathing. This can be accomplished by reassuring the victim, instructing him or her in deep diaphragmatic breathing, and breathing in through the nose and out through the mouth. Breathing into a paper bag is not recommended because it can decrease oxygen levels and lead to hypoxia. Additional support for

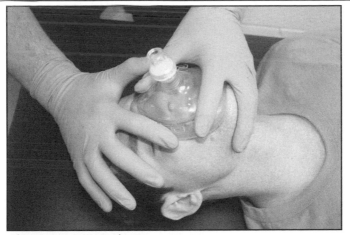

Figure 4-9. CPR mask.

Figure 4-10. Bag-valve mask.

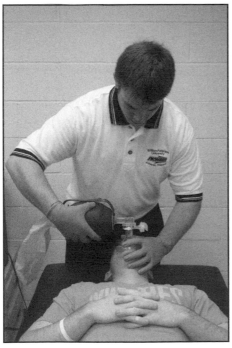

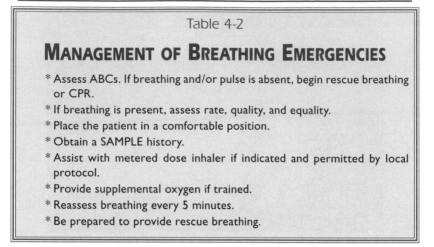

Table 4-2

MANAGEMENT OF BREATHING EMERGENCIES

* Assess ABCs. If breathing and/or pulse is absent, begin rescue breathing or CPR.
* If breathing is present, assess rate, quality, and equality.
* Place the patient in a comfortable position.
* Obtain a SAMPLE history.
* Assist with metered dose inhaler if indicated and permitted by local protocol.
* Provide supplemental oxygen if trained.
* Reassess breathing every 5 minutes.
* Be prepared to provide rescue breathing.

breathing includes placing the patient in a position of comfort and loosening any restrictive clothing. Patients who are experiencing difficulty breathing may feel most comfortable in the tripod position (seated forward with elbows on knees). The sports emergency care provider should continue to perform a detailed physical examination, as well as obtain a SAMPLE history. If the patient has a prescription for medication to assist breathing (such as for asthma), assist him or her in administering the medication if local protocol allows (Table 4-2).

OXYGEN ADMINISTRATION

The use of oxygen in emergency situations is beneficial because it increases the concentration of oxygen inhaled and aids in the prevention and management of hypoxia and shock. For EMTs and paramedics, the use of supplemental oxygen is standard practice for treatment of suddenly ill or injured victims. However, while the use of oxygen is a skill routinely performed by EMS professionals, there has been some debate as to whether athletic trainers can administer oxygen. Athletic trainers can, in fact, administer oxygen in emergency situations.

The Food and Drug Administration (FDA) classifies oxygen as a drug, and as such containers used to store oxygen (the oxygen tank) are subject to specific regulations. Oxygen equipment is divided into 2 categories: therapeutic oxygen and emergency oxygen (Figure 4-11). In both categories, the gas is the same; it is the method of delivery that differs. Therapeutic oxygen systems such as those commonly found in hospitals and ambulances may only be operated by allied health and medical personnel licensed to do so and only

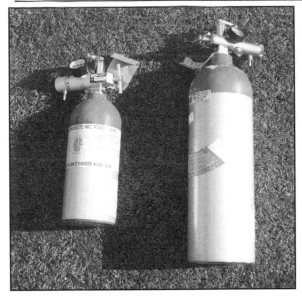

Figure 4-11. Oxygen delivery systems.

if authorized by a prescription from a licensed physician. Therapeutic oxygen delivery systems must include a container suitable for holding medical grade oxygen, a pressure-reducing system (often called a regulator), a contents indicator such as a gauge, and some means of delivering oxygen to the patient such as through the use of a mask or cannula. Therapeutic oxygen delivery systems are able to deliver oxygen at a flow rate of less than 6 L per minute (Lpm) and last less than 15 minutes.

Like therapeutic oxygen delivery systems, emergency oxygen delivery systems include a container, pressure-reducing system, gauge, and a patient delivery system (mask). However, there are 2 main differences between emergency and therapeutic oxygen systems (Table 4-3). Emergency oxygen delivery systems must be capable of delivering oxygen at a flow rate of at least 6 Lpm for at least 15 minutes. Furthermore, emergency oxygen delivery systems are available over the counter and may be obtained without prescription. Anyone who has received proper training in the use of emergency oxygen, including athletic trainers, may use it when providing emergency care to an ill or injured person.

Conclusion

Establishing and maintaining a patent airway should always be the primary concern when treating a suddenly ill or injured athlete. Regardless of the nature of the injury or illness, the lack of a patent airway can lead to

Table 4-3

DIFFERENCES BETWEEN THERAPEUTIC AND EMERGENCY OXYGEN SYSTEMS

Therapeutic Oxygen	Emergency Oxygen
Has a container holding medical grade oxygen Has a pressure-reducing system Has a contents indicator (gauge) Uses a mask or other means to deliver oxygen	
Able to deliver oxygen at a flow rate of less than 6 Lpm or lasts less than 15 minutes	Delivers oxygen at a flow rate of at least 6 Lpm for at least 15 minutes
Delivers oxygen via an adjustable flow regulator	Delivers oxygen at a fixed flow rate
Prescription required for use	Available over the counter without prescription

respiratory compromise, respiratory arrest, and even death. Sports emergency care personnel should be proficient in airway management and the use of airway adjuncts, as well as possess the ability to recognize and treat breathing emergencies.

Bibliography

American Heart Association. 2005 American Heart Association guidelines for cardiopulmonary resuscitation and emergency cardiovascular care. Circulation. November 28, 2005. Available at: http://circ.ahajournals.org/cgi/content/full/112/24_suppl/IV-1. Accessed July 2, 2006.

National Highway Traffic Safety Administration. EMT-Basic: national standard curriculum. Available at: http://www.nhtsa.dot.gov/people/injury/ems/pub/emtbnsc.pdf. Accessed November 2, 2006.

National Safety Council. *Oxygen Administration*. Boston, Mass: Jones and Bartlett Publishers; 1995.

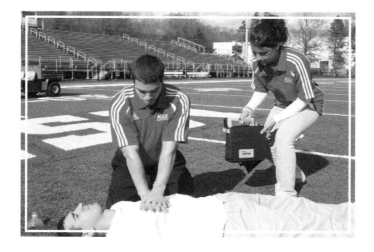

Chapter **5**   # Cardiovascular Emergencies

Robb S. Rehberg, PhD, ATC, CSCS, NREMT

Of all the possible injuries and illnesses with which sports emergency care personnel are faced, cardiovascular emergencies can be the most challenging. Prompt recognition of signs and symptoms of cardiovascular emergencies followed by rapid intervention can mean the difference between life and death. While most athletes are generally healthy and do not fit the profile of individuals at risk for cardiovascular disease and related conditions such as heart attack and stroke, they are not immune to these types of conditions. Moreover, other cardiovascular conditions such as underlying congenital heart defects, trauma, and other cardiovascular disorders do occur in sports.

Sports emergency care personnel must anticipate cardiovascular emergencies and be prepared to quickly manage these conditions. All sports emergency care personnel should be trained in CPR for health care professionals and be proficient in resuscitative skills.

Review of Clinically Relevant Anatomy

The heart is the central organ in the cardiovascular system. It is positioned centrally in the thoracic cavity. It lies obliquely between the lungs. One-third of the heart is posterior to the sternum; the remainder lies to the left of the sternum.

The heart is a muscular organ composed of 4 chambers. It is enclosed by the pericardium. The upper chambers are the 2 atria. The lower chambers are the 2 ventricles. The atria are separated by a partition called the interatrial septum. The ventricles are separated by the interventricular septum. There are 4 valves in the heart to ensure proper flow of blood through the 4 chambers of the heart and connecting great vessels. The blood supply to the heart muscle itself is supplied by the coronary arteries.

The flow of blood through the heart starts in the right atrium. The right atrium receives deoxygenated blood from the superior vena cava, the inferior vena cava, and the coronary sinus. From the right atrium, blood flows through the tricuspid valve, into the right ventricle. The right ventricle pumps blood into the right and left pulmonary arteries, which carries blood to the lungs, where it is oxygenated. Blood returns to the heart via the pulmonary veins, which empty into the left atrium. From the left atrium, blood flows through the mitral valve into the left ventricle. The left ventricle pumps blood out of the heart through the aortic valve into the ascending aorta. The ascending aorta becomes the arch of the aorta, then the thoracic aorta, and then the abdominal aorta. These vessels supply blood to the rest of the body.

Assessment of Chest Pain

Sports emergency care personnel must pay particular attention to the athlete who presents with chest pain or chest discomfort. While chest pain is often considered a cardinal sign of a cardiac-related event, chest pain can present as a result of several factors, some cardiac related and others of noncardiac origin. Any athlete who presents with chest pain, regardless of age or fitness level, should be assessed thoroughly to rule out a cardiac-related illness. Additionally, while chest "pain" is the most common descriptor of the sensation in the chest as a result of a cardiac-related event, some patients experiencing a cardiac-related event may use other descriptors such as discomfort, pressure, ache, burning, or fullness rather than pain.[1] Therefore, sports emergency care personnel should treat chest discomfort that is unrelated to trauma as a cardiac-related event until proven otherwise. Noncardiac-related chest pain can often be explained due to obvious injury, mechanism of injury, or recent illness. Other causes may be more difficult to determine. Table 5-1 lists examples of cardiac versus noncardiac-related chest pain.

Sudden Cardiac Arrest in Sports

Sudden cardiac arrest (SCA), also known as sudden cardiac death, is defined as the sudden, abrupt loss of heart function in a person who may or may not have diagnosed heart disease.[2] It is the leading cause of death in young athletes.[3] Loss of heart function can occur as a result of many factors, both atraumatic, including hypertrophic cardiomyopathy and other congenital heart abnormalities, and traumatic, as in the case of commotio cordis.

HYPERTROPHIC CARDIOMYOPATHY

Hypertrophic cardiomyopathy is the leading cause of sudden cardiac death among young athletes. According to a study by Maron et al, hypertrophic cardiomyopathy and cases suspected to be hypertrophic cardiomyopathy account

Table 5-1

COMMON CAUSES OF CHEST PAIN

Cardiac	Noncardiac
Myocardial infarction	Gastroesophageal reflux disease
Angina	Esophagitis
Hypertrophic cardiomyopathy	Esophageal spasm
Aortic stenosis	Ulcers
Cardiac tamponade	Asthma
Cardiac contusion	Gastritis
Coronary artery disorders	Pneumothorax
Valve disorders	Pulmonary embolism
Aortic dissection	Pleuritis
	Bronchitis
	Costochondral injury
	Rib fracture
	Herpes zoster

for nearly half of all cases of sudden cardiac death.[3] Hypertrophic cardiomyopathy is a congenital heart defect characterized by an abnormal enlargement or thickening of the left ventricular wall of the heart in the absence of a cardiac or systemic condition that produces left ventricular hypertrophy. It is estimated that hypertrophic cardiomyopathy affects 1 in 500 people.[4] Many athletes with hypertrophic cardiomyopathy are often asymptomatic, with the first presenting sign being SCA. Therefore, sports emergency care personnel must be prepared to provide resuscitation at any time. Some athletes may present with cardiac-related symptoms on exertion, such as chest discomfort, shortness of breath, and syncope, so it is important that sports emergency care personnel conduct a thorough assessment on any athlete presenting with signs and symptoms that may be of cardiac origin.

COMMOTIO CORDIS

Commotio cordis, which literally means "concussion of the heart," is defined as sudden cardiac death that occurs as a result of a blow to the chest. It is caused when the blow to the chest occurs during the vulnerable repolarization phase of the cardiac electrical cycle (15 milliseconds to 30 milliseconds prior to the T wave). Commotio cordis occurs most often in children due to the pliability of the chest wall. Although the occurrence of sudden cardiac death due to commotio cordis is relatively low, researchers speculate that this cause of death may be underreported.

Commotio cordis can be caused by a direct blow to the chest by an object such as a baseball or hockey puck or from being struck in the chest by an opponent through physical contact, as in martial arts. When commotio cordis occurs, the athlete usually collapses within seconds of the blow to the chest, although a brief moment of continued activity may be observed prior to the sudden collapse. The athlete will present as unresponsive, apneic, and pulseless. The survival rate for victims of commotio cordis is approximately 15%.[5] Victims of commotio cordis have the best chance of survival when CPR and defibrillation are administered immediately.

Management of Sudden Cardiac Arrest

In August 2006, the National Athletic Trainers' Association convened an Inter-Association Task Force for Emergency Preparedness and Management of Sudden Cardiac Arrest in High School and College Athletic Programs. This multidisciplinary group consisted of representatives from 15 national professional organizations. The Task Force recommends the following steps be taken for the management of SCA[6]:

- Management begins with appropriate emergency preparedness, CPR and AED training for all likely first responders, and access to early defibrillation.

- Essential components of SCA management include early activation of EMS, early CPR, early defibrillation, and rapid transition to advanced cardiac life support.

- High suspicion of SCA should be maintained for any collapsed and unresponsive athlete.

- SCA in athletes can be mistaken for other causes of collapse. Rescuers should be trained to recognize SCA in athletes with special focus on potential barriers to recognizing SCA, including inaccurate rescuer assessment of pulse or respirations, occasional or agonal gasping, and myoclonic or seizure-like activity.

- Young athletes who collapse shortly after being struck in the chest by a firm projectile or by contact with another player should be suspected of having SCA from a condition known as commotio cordis.

- Any collapsed and unresponsive athlete should be managed as a SCA with application of an AED as soon as possible for rhythm analysis and defibrillation, if indicated.

- CPR should be provided while waiting for an AED.

- Interruptions in chest compressions should be minimized and CPR stopped only for rhythm analysis and shock.

- CPR should be resumed immediately after the first shock, beginning with chest compressions, with repeat rhythm analysis following 2 minutes or 5 cycles of CPR, or until advanced life support providers take over or the victim starts to move.
- Rapid access to the SCA victim should be facilitated for EMS personnel.

Other Common Cardiovascular Emergencies

MYOCARDIAL INFARCTION

Myocardial infarction, otherwise known as a heart attack, can occur in any athletic setting. Although athletic trainers often work with athletes in generally good health, sports emergency care personnel must be prepared to manage myocardial infarction in athletes, coaches, officials, or others. Myocardial infarction occurs when there is a decrease in oxygenated blood flow to the heart muscle due to a blockage of a coronary artery. Signs and symptoms of myocardial infarction may be overt, with classic chest pain and associated signs and symptoms including profuse sweating (diaphoresis), difficulty breathing, respiratory difficulty, nausea, and dizziness. Pain may also radiate to the neck, jaw, arms (the left arm is more common), and back. As discussed earlier, some patients may not complain of pain but of pressure or ache. Thus, it is important for the sports emergency care personnel to perform a thorough assessment.

Sports emergency care personnel should manage an individual experiencing signs and symptoms of myocardial infarction by performing a thorough assessment, placing the victim in a position of comfort (usually in a reclining position), and loosening any restrictive clothing. High-flow oxygen should be administered if available, and EMS should be activated immediately. Sports emergency care personnel should continuously monitor vital signs and be prepared to provide resuscitation or defibrillation if the victim's condition deteriorates to cardiac arrest.

ANGINA PECTORIS

Angina pectoris is a transient chest pain that results when the heart's demand for oxygenated blood exceeds supply from the coronary arteries. This decrease in oxygenated blood supply is usually caused by coronary artery spasm. Signs and symptoms of angina pectoris are similar to that of myocardial infarction. The main difference in the sports setting is that most athletes who present with angina pectoris will have already been diagnosed with the condition. Patients diagnosed with angina pectoris are often prescribed nitroglycerine to be used when symptoms occur. If permitted by local protocol and properly trained, sports emergency care personnel should assist patients in the administration of their prescribed nitroglycerine medication as directed. If symptoms do not resolve with medication or if symptoms become worse, provide similar care for that of a patient presenting with a myocardial infarction.

STROKE

Incidence of stroke is rare in sports. Stroke (also known as cerebrovascular accident) is defined as a decrease in oxygenated blood flow to the brain. Stroke is commonly classified by the cause of the decrease in oxygenated blood. Ischemic stroke, the most common form, occurs when an artery carrying blood to the brain is blocked. Causes of blockage include a narrowing of the arteries (atherosclerosis) and a blood clot (thrombus or embolus). Hemorrhagic stroke occurs when an artery carrying blood to the brain ruptures, either due to traumatic injury or as a result of an aneurysm that has ruptured.

Signs and symptoms of stroke include sudden numbness; decrease or loss of function of the face, arm, or leg, usually affecting only one side of the body; sudden severe headache; vision disturbances; unequal pupils; loss of balance or coordination; mental confusion; difficulty speaking or swallowing; or loss of bowel and bladder control.

Sports emergency care personnel should provide immediate care for the stroke patient by protecting the airway, assessing vital signs, performing a detailed history and physical exam, and administering high flow oxygen, if trained. Patients exhibiting signs and symptoms of stroke should be transported by EMS to the nearest hospital immediately. Recent advances in the treatment of ischemic stroke can often provide the patient with a favorable prognosis if treatment is initiated immediately.

CARDIAC TAMPONADE

Cardiac tamponade is a compression of the heart caused by a collection of blood or fluid in the pericardial sac. The pericardial sac is an inelastic membrane that surrounds the heart. If blood collects rapidly between the heart and pericardium from a cardiac injury, the ventricles are compressed. It is most often associated with penetrating chest trauma and is rare in sports. Cardiac tamponade can be fatal if not recognized and treated immediately. Even a small amount of pericardial blood may compromise cardiac function. As the compression of the ventricles increases, the heart is less able to refill and cardiac output decreases.

Clinical presentation of cardiac tamponade includes signs and symptoms of shock, as well as hypotension, jugular vein distention, and muffled heart sounds. Muffled heart sounds may be difficult to hear at some sports venues due to the noise level. The athlete may have a paradoxical pulse. If the athlete loses his or her peripheral pulse during inspiration, this is suggestive of a paradoxical pulse and the presence of cardiac tamponade. The major differential diagnosis in the field is tension pneumothorax. However, unlike a pneumothorax, the patient with cardiac tamponade will present with a midline trachea (as opposed to tracheal deviation) and equal breath sounds unless there is an associated pneumothorax or hemothorax.

TRAUMATIC AORTIC RUPTURE

Traumatic aortic rupture is a very rare injury in sports and is most common in motor vehicle accidents and falls from great heights. The vast majority of patients die immediately. For those who survive, fast proper diagnosis is essential because emergency surgery is necessary for survival. Traumatic thoracic aortic tears are usually due to deceleration injury with the heart and aortic arch moving suddenly anteriorly, transecting the aorta. In the patients who do not exsanguinate quickly, the surrounding tissue may temporarily contain the aortic tear and limit bleeding.

The diagnosis of a contained thoracic aortic laceration is extremely difficult, especially in the field. Sports emergency care providers should consider mechanism of injury since victims of aortic lacerations often show no outward signs of chest trauma. In rare cases, the athlete may present with upper extremity hypertension and diminished pulses in the lower extremity.

MYOCARDIAL CONTUSION

Myocardial contusion is a potentially life-threatening injury that can occur in contact sports from a blunt trauma chest injury. Blunt injury to the anterior chest is transmitted via the sternum to the heart, which lies immediately posterior. Cardiac injuries from this mechanism may also include valve rupture, pericardial tamponade, or cardiac rupture. Due to the position of the heart, contusions to the right atrium and right ventricle occur more commonly than those to the left atrium and left ventricle. A victim with a myocardial contusion will present with similar signs and symptoms as in an acute myocardial infarction, including chest pain, dysrhythmia, or cardiogenic shock. In the field, cardiogenic shock may not be distinguishable from cardiac tamponade. Chest pain may be difficult to differentiate from the associated musculoskeletal discomfort (sternal contusion, rib contusion/fracture) that the athlete may suffer as a result of the injury.

CARDIAC ARRHYTHMIAS

Abnormal heart electrophysiology can produce arrhythmias that have the potential to cause cardiovascular emergencies. They can reduce cardiac output, impairing perfusion of the myocardium or the brain and causing myocardial infarction or a syncopal or near-syncopal episode. Cardiac arrhythmias can sometimes be detected during preparticipation physical examination (PPPE); however, they are often detected only after signs and symptoms of a cardiac event have occurred.

There are many types of arrhythmias and treatment plans will vary, as will clearance for level of physical activity. While arrhythmias among young athletes are usually benign, they raise concern due to the heightened awareness of sudden death that has been attributed to cardiac conditions. Many common arrhythmias such as Wolff Parkinson White and Long QT syndromes may not be symptomatic. When symptomatic, signs and symptoms of a cardiac arrhythmia may include palpitations, syncope, near syncope, dizziness, fatigue, or sudden death.

MYOCARDITIS

Myocarditis is an inflammation of the myocardium caused by infection. Common signs and symptoms of myocarditis can include cough, shortness of breath, and chest pain, all of which intensify with exercise. Athletes with myocarditis will likely exhibit flu-like symptoms, including body ache, joint pain, headache, sore throat, fever, and diarrhea. Myocarditis may be difficult to detect in the field due to the accompanying flu-like symptoms. Athletes with myocarditis risk developing a fatal arrhythmia upon exertion, further reinforcing the need for careful medical evaluation for any athlete exhibiting possible signs of cardiac nature.

SYNCOPE

A common cause of syncope is due to a decrease of oxygenated blood to the brain. This condition can be benign, such as syncope due to emotional distress or orthostatic hypotension. However, syncope can also be an indicator of cardiac insufficiency. Sports emergency care personnel should conduct a thorough assessment on any athlete who loses consciousness and consider all possible causes. Additional information on syncope is included in Chapter 7.

VALVE AND BLOOD VESSEL DISORDERS

Other conditions related to valve defects such as aortic stenosis, aortic regurgitation, mitral valve stenosis, and mitral valve regurgitation have the potential to produce a cardiac event upon exertion. Additionally, blood vessel disorders such as aortic aneurysm and aortic dissection can cause SCA upon exertion. These conditions may be difficult, if not impossible, to detect in the field unless revealed by the patient while obtaining medical history.

Conclusion

There are many cardiovascular conditions that affect athletes. Some conditions are benign and do not pose a threat while participating in physical activity. Others can be fatal if untreated or undetected. Still other traumatic events can cause sudden cardiac death in athletes. While there can be many causes of chest pain and sudden cardiac death in athletes, sports emergency care personnel must take great care in recognizing potential cardiac-related events and must be prepared to provide resuscitative efforts at any time.

References

1. Bahr RD, Christenson RH, Farin H, et al. Prodromal symptoms of acute myocardial infarction: overview of evidence. *Med Ed J.* 2001;106-108.

2. American Heart Association. Sudden cardiac death. Available at: http://www. americanheart.org/presenter.jhtml?identifier=14. Accessed September 14, 2006.

3. Maron BJ, Shirani J, Poliac LC, Mathenge R, Roberts WC, Mueller FO. Sudden death in young competitive athletes: clinical, demographic, and pathological profiles. *JAMA.* 1996;276:199-204.

4. Maron BJ. Hypertrophic cardiomyopathy: a systemic review. *JAMA.* 2002;287:1308-1320.

5. Maron BJ, Gohman TE, Kyle SB, Estes NA, Link MS. Clinical profile and spectrum of commotio cordis. *JAMA.* 2002;287:1142-1146.

6. Courson RW, Drezner, J. Consensus statement: inter-association task force recommendations on emergency preparedness and management of sudden cardiac arrest in high school and college athletic programs. Available at: http://www. nata.org/statements/consensus/sca_executive_summary.pdf. Accessed November 22, 2006.

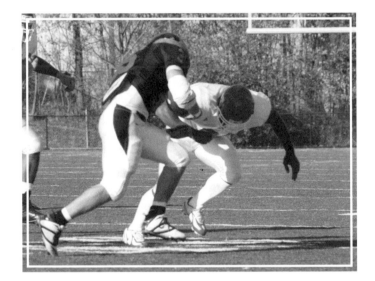

Management of Spinal Injuries

Chapter **6**

Michael J. Cendoma, MS, ATC and Robb S. Rehberg, PhD, ATC, CSCS, NREMT

There is no way to express the range of emotions that will be experienced when one is confronted with a critically injured athlete. In a single instant, the athlete is transformed from a competitive athlete into a critically injured person; a critically injured person who is someone's child. It is at this instant that a sports health care professional will first see ultimate fear in an injured person's eyes and will feel this ultimate fear in the hearts of the injured athlete's family, friends, and teammates. It is at this moment that the sports health care professional realizes that prior preparation, practice, and mental rehearsal can mean the difference between a person living or dying, between a person walking away from a serious injury or living life with a devastating disability. It is only at this exact moment that a sports health care professional will truly come to realize what it means to be responsible for the care and management of athletic injuries and how vital it is to be able to rely on psychomotor skills and an EAP that have been practiced so frequently that they have become second nature.

This chapter is a pragmatic discussion regarding the emergency management objectives and psychomotor skills that every sports emergency care team must be able to demonstrate during the care and management of the athlete with a potential cervical spine injury (CSI). Injuries to the thoracic and lumbar spine also occur in athletics and require use of proper spine injury precautions during management. However, we will focus on injuries involving the cervical spine because they are the most prevalent and devastating spinal injuries in athletics. This chapter will provide a brief overview of mechanisms of injury and neurophysiology as a basis for understanding the practical discussion regarding acute assessment of an athlete with a CSI. The chapter will also address proper transfer of an athlete with a potential CSI to a rigid immobilization device and proper preparation of the immobilized athlete for transport to an appropriate medical facility. Finally, ER management, including initial radiographic assessment of the potentially spine-injured athlete, will also be discussed.

Spinal injuries can result from participation in any sport. However, this chapter's emphasis is on equipment-intensive sports such as football, lacrosse, and hockey due to the unique challenges that this protective equipment presents to sports emergency care team members during injury management. Regardless of the sport and type of protective equipment in use, the single-most effective strategy for successful injury management begins with a sound EAP based on a sports emergency care team approach.

Only those EAPs that incorporate regular rehearsal and are designed around a sports emergency care team approach provide sports health care professionals with any opportunity to mediate the outcome of a critically injured athlete. As discussed earlier, development and implementation of an EAP must involve the coordinated efforts of certified athletic trainers, EMS, ER personnel, coaches, and school officials.

Mechanism of Injury

When caring for an athlete with a potential CSI, the foremost sign or symptom that warrants a conservative on-field assessment by the effective sports emergency care team is the mechanism of injury. Consideration of the mechanism of injury is an important first step in the on-field assessment of any athletic injury; however, perhaps in no other injury situation is initial determination of the mechanism of injury as vital as in the care of an athlete with a potential CSI. Failure to identify the mechanism of injury associated with a CSI could lead to major disability or death resulting from improper acute care. An athlete having suffered a significant CSI may not immediately present with the obvious neurological signs and symptoms so often associated with CSI, though more subtle signs and symptoms of underlying spinal trauma will be present. Therefore, the mechanism of injury alone indicates the need to carefully assess an athlete with a potential CSI for the presence of the obvious and subtler signs and symptoms in order to render appropriate acute care for the athlete. The axial loading mechanism of injury is the most widely publicized mechanism of CSI in athletics.[1]

Axial Loading

The axial loading mechanism of injury accounts for between 8 and 13 catastrophic cervical spine injuries annually in football.[2] The most disturbing aspect of CSI resulting from axial loading is that it is often avoidable. Too frequently, these injuries are brought about by a conscious effort to use the crown of the head as the initial point of contact or as a result of improper technique. Equally disturbing is that some are still inclined to present these injuries as

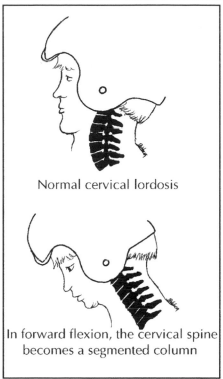

Normal cervical lordosis

In forward flexion, the cervical spine becomes a segmented column

Figure 6-1. Axial loading. (Illustration by Joelle Rehberg, DO.)

"freak" accidents.[3,4] The physics of axial loading and its relationship to CSI are well documented. There is no such thing as a "freak" CSI. Athletes who place themselves in positions known to be associated with CSI run a higher risk of CSI and paralysis. Covering these injuries with the "freak" accident blanket only minimizes the importance of coaching and using proper technique.[5] The "freak" accident blanket also allows others to play under the false pretense that these injuries are total random occurrences. Sports health care professionals must understand axial loading in order to be able to recognize it on-field and to be able to clearly demonstrate to others that, in the majority of cases, intentional or unintentional head-down contact results in CSI in football.[6]

The cervical spine possesses a natural lordotic curve when erect. The normal lordotic curve of the cervical spine is lost when a person's head is in a head-down position, resulting in a straight segmented vertebral column (Figure 6-1). The normal cervical lordotic curve is vital in helping the surrounding soft tissue absorb and dissipate energy through deformation and bending. When in a head-down position, the vertebral column is in the straight segmented position. Contact with the top of the head when the cervical spine is in a straight segmented position results in kinetic energy being transferred to the vertebral column as strain energy. When strain energy exceeds the absorbing capabilities of the column, the result is failure in the form of intervertebral disk space injury, vertebral body fracture, disruption of ligamentous and other soft tissues, or posterior element fracture. The location at which vertebral failure occurs becomes the unstable segment in the column. Further compressive force produces a large angulation or hyperflexion as a means of releasing the additional strain energy. Hyperflexion at the failed vertebral level produces dislocation of the unstable segment, resulting in major neurological damage.

The compressive load limits or energy required to produce failure of a vertebral segment have been calculated to be between 3340 Newton (N) and 4450 N. These limits are easily reached when the head is lowered and used as the initial point of contact.[7] In fact, when contact is made at the apex or anterior to the apex of the helmet while in a head-down position, the compressive load limits of the cervical vertebral column are reached within 11 milliseconds of impact. The rapidness with which the compressive load limits of the cervical vertebral column are reached has 2 major implications in resulting injury to the cervical spine. First, at the same time that compressive load limits within the cervical vertebra are being reached, the compressive force being applied to the cervical spine is continuing to increase due to the athlete's torso continuing to accelerate forward after the head decelerated upon impact. The continued force applied by the torso results in the cervical spine being exposed to compressive forces that cause hyperflexion, resulting in dislocation of unstable vertebral segments. A second important implication resulting from the rapidness with which compressive load limits are reached in the cervical spine is that 11 milliseconds is not enough time for reflex-mediated muscle contraction. Reflex-mediated muscle contraction occurs at 60 milliseconds, which is not enough time for the musculature of the neck to provide any resistance to the hyperflexion caused by continued force from the oncoming torso.[1,8]

Understanding of the axial loading mechanism led the National Collegiate Athletic Association (NCAA) and the National Federation of High Schools to institute rule changes regarding using the head as the initial point of contact, or spearing, in 1976. Proper technique and adherence to rule changes initiated as a result of the clinical findings relating to spearing, either intentional or unintentional, could prevent many of the cervical spine injuries in football. Still, it appears that spearing is as prevalent now as it was prior to the 1976 rule changes.[9] Sports health care professionals should educate players, coaches, and officials that head-down contact, either intentional or unintentional, increases the likelihood of suffering a CSI in football. Coaches should increase the time athletes spend practicing proper techniques that keep the head out of contact while officials should strive to enforce rules regarding involvement of the head in contact. The education of athletes, prudent coaching, and rule enforcement would likely reduce the incidence of head-down contact, thus reducing the possibility of axial loading and catastrophic CSI in football.[6]

Although axial loading accounts for 52% of the cervical spine injuries in football, 48% result from some other mechanism of injury.[10,11] CSI occurs in sports other than football as well. To discuss only axial loading in football would suggest that cervical spine injuries only occur as a result of axial loading during football season. Discussing axial loading only would also suggest that only those signs and symptoms associated with major neurological complications resulting from fracture and dislocation of cervical vertebral segments during an axial load would comprise a sufficient on-field assessment. Cervical spine injuries happen in all sports and result from other mechanisms of injury that may or may not present with the immediate signs and symptoms associated with major neurological complications. In fact, movement of the head and neck in any plane could be a mechanism of injury, particularly when the movement is excessive or rapid in nature.[8] Therefore, the sports emergency care team must be prepared to conduct a thorough on-field assessment with CSI precautions any time a possible injury to the cervical spine involves hyperflexion, hyperextension, lateral bending, or rotation.

Neurophysiology

CSI resulting in severe neurological deficit may not be associated with injury to the vertebral column. In fact, the neural tissues remain intact in most spinal cord injury cases. Within 30 min to 60 min after trauma, an autodestructive process referred to as spinal shock is initiated within the spinal cord. Spinal shock is characterized by mechanical, biochemical, and hemodynamic changes that bring about an ischemic or hypoxic state within the cells of neural tissues. Once initiated, these changes facilitate one another, leading to a worsening progression that has been reported to lead to necrosis involving up to 40% of the cross-sectional gray matter area within 4 hours of insult.[12,13]

Spinal shock has profound and lasting effects on all body systems. An understanding of spinal shock and its role in determining the extent of injury is an important aspect of acute spinal cord injury care and recovery. The importance of the sports emergency care team approach to acute prehospital care is emphasized throughout this text. Considering that the effects of spinal shock can take hold in as little as 30 minutes and can lead to significant neural tissue loss within 4 hours, the sports emergency care team must operate efficiently. In most instances, assessment, immobilization, and transfer of the athlete with a potential CSI to an ER are not time-consuming processes. However, injured neural tissue requires very specific acute care that is not readily available in any hospital ER. Therefore, it is important for the sports emergency care team to work efficiently in assessing, immobilizing, and transporting the athlete to the hospital and for the team to include local ER personnel. This arrangement will give the athlete the best chance for proper initial on-field management, timely diagnosis, and quick transfer to a neural trauma center.

SPINAL SHOCK CASCADE

Spinal shock affects the spinal cord and neural tissues in 2 stages that can be identified as the primary and secondary phases of injury.

The primary injury phase of spinal shock involves actual structural damage to the neural tissues.[14] The primary injury is due to a mechanical insult, such as a vertebral fracture, subluxation, dislocation, intervertebral disk disruption, or pressure gradient changes. The spinal cord's initial response to a mechanical insult is hemorrhage, vacuolation, and swelling of capillary endothelium.[13] The extent of neural tissue injury is proportional to the force associated with the mechanical insult, affecting an area referred to as the zone of injury. Although less than 10% of the spinal cord provides for locomotion, the zone of injury can increase in less than 30 minutes due to the cascading complications of spinal shock typical in the secondary injury phase.[12-14] In order to restrict the zone of injury to that area affected by the initial mechanical insult, the sports emergency care team must recognize the subtle signs and symptoms indicating the presence of spinal shock and effectively care for the acutely injured athlete during the primary injury phase. Signs and symptoms indicating the presence of spinal shock may be immediately identified by the presence of hypotension, bradycardia, and loss of reflexes.[12]

The secondary injury phase has been characterized as a pathophysiologic cascade of injury initiated shortly after the primary injury. Ischemia is the dominant component of this phase, resulting from a decrease in the autoregulatory response of neural vasculature that can result in a significant reduction in blood flow to the spinal cord within 2 hours. Ischemia, the progression of edema, and an autodestructive biochemical process are serious complications associated with the secondary injury phase. Edema may first be observed at the injury site during the primary injury phase, but quickly spreads during the secondary injury phase. The net result of the secondary injury phase can be an autodestructive cascade of events that result in ischemia, cell death, and permanent neurological damage.[12,14]

Acute Management of Spinal Injuries

Acute on-field management can have a significant impact on the extent of secondary injury suffered by athletes with spinal injuries.[15,16] Improved equipment, better safety techniques, and a more efficient EMS system decrease the time required to transfer spine-injured athletes to spinal cord trauma facilities and decrease the extent of neurological deficit at admission.[17] Thus, a team approach that incorporates the best equipment, techniques, and organized personnel provides the best chance for preventing secondary injury and can significantly improve a patient's prognosis for recovery.[17] The importance of sports health care professionals working together as part of an effective sports emergency care team approach to effective on-field management of an athlete with a potential CSI is undisputed.[12,18,19]

Acute on-field management of the athlete with a potential spine injury begins with the sports emergency care team conducting a primary injury assessment for immediate life-threatening injuries. A primary assessment is conducted to assess the athlete's airway, breathing, circulation, severe bleeding, shock, and spinal injury (ABC Sx3). Three unique considerations must be taken into account when conducting a primary survey on an athlete with a potential CSI. First, upon determining a mechanism of injury that could involve the cervical spine, the sports emergency care team must immediately immobilize the athlete's head and neck in the position in which the athlete is found. Repositioning the athlete's head and neck is contraindicated as long as there are no immediate concerns regarding airway, breathing, and circulation. The athlete will eventually be repositioned into inline stabilization either later in the secondary assessment or when transferred to a rigid support for transport by EMS. The first team member to reach the athlete immobilizes the head and neck. The sports health care professional immobilizing the supine athlete's head and neck should place his or her hands such that the palms face each other. The hands are then slid along the side of the athlete's head and neck until the web space of the sports health care professional's thumb meets the base of the athlete's neck. The professional's arms are then positioned on the lateral aspects of the athlete's head and neck so as to prevent as much motion as possible within the head and neck complex (Figure 6-2). The team member immobilizing the head and neck should then rest his or her forearms on his or her thighs with his or her back kept straight. Positioning of the individual immobilizing the head and neck is important because the immobilization of the athlete's head and neck may have to be maintained for an extended period of time. Discomfort or injury to the sports health care provider due to poor ergonomics could result in unnecessary movement of the injured athlete when the sports health care professional is forced to reposition him- or herself or transfer immobilization of the injured athlete's head and neck.

A second unique consideration that must be considered when planning the care of an athlete with a potential CSI is that the sports emergency care team must gain immediate control over the injury scene, particularly being able to ensure that the athlete remains still and cooperative during the assessment process. Finally, the sports emergency care team must be more sensitive to subtle abnormalities when assessing an athlete's vital signs. Careful assessment and interpretation of the athlete's vital signs may provide important clues regarding the presence of spinal shock when more obvious signs and symptoms of spinal injury are not present. The following section details specific signs and

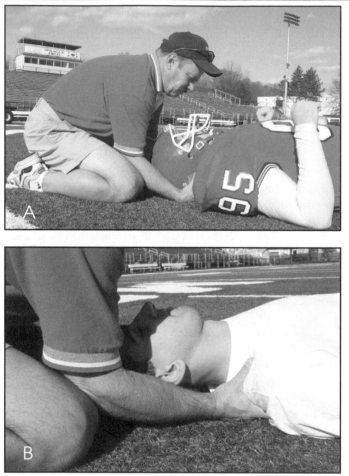

Figure 6-2. Spinal stabilization techniques.

symptoms of underlying spinal shock that can be observed when assessing the athlete's vital signs when conducting a primary injury assessment.

PRIMARY INJURY ASSESSMENT

The primary injury assessment of an athlete with a potential CSI begins with an assessment of the athlete's airway, breathing, and circulation. The efficient sports emergency care team is able to render emergency care for an athlete's vitals signs while taking precautions to protect the cervical spine. The following discussion pertaining to the primary injury assessment will review assessment of an athlete with a potential CSI and spinal shock. Special consideration is given to athletes in protective equipment and spine injury precautions when relevant.

Airway

The critical components of airway maintenance include ensuring an open and clear airway. The sports emergency care team should not rely on the conventional head-tilt chin-lift technique as an initial means of opening a compromised airway because hyperextension within the cervical region associated with the head-tilt chin-lift maneuver could cause unstable vertebrae to intrude on the vertebral canal. As little as 1 mm of movement within the cervical vertebral column could increase the risk of further injury to the athlete.[18] The well-equipped and prepared sports emergency care team is prepared to avoid the head-tilt chin-lift maneuver by making use of alternative techniques such as the modified jaw thrust or chin-tilt maneuver. The modified jaw thrust is performed by lifting the chin without tilting the head. If this technique is not successful in establishing an airway, an advanced airway technique should be used so as to avoid the dangers associated with the head-tilt chin-lift maneuver. Using an advanced airway technique on an athlete in a protective helmet may first require facemask extraction. Facemask removal will be covered in detail when discussing breathing assessment and care (see pp. 81-83).

The jaw thrust and advanced airway techniques are particularly challenging to perform on an athlete in a protective helmet. Therefore, the sports emergency care team must practice these techniques on athletes in protective gear to ensure that sports emergency care team personnel have the psychomotor skills required to perform these tasks in an emergency. The sports emergency care team can assess the athlete's breathing status once the athlete's airway has been established.

Breathing

During the initial assessment of the athlete's breathing, the sports emergency care team will be confronted with one of the following situations: the athlete is breathing well enough on his or her own, the athlete is not breathing, or the rate and tidal volume of breathing is insufficient to support vital body function.

Breathing, or respiration, rates that are sufficient in the athlete with a potential CSI may be disrupted as a result of a somewhat likely chance that a CSI athlete will vomit. Therefore, suction should be available and immediately administered with the onset of vomiting to prevent disruption of the flow of oxygen.[20] Clearing the airway of vomit without suction will prove much more challenging, particularly following immobilization of the athlete to a rigid support.

In the absence of vomit or other foreign airway obstructions that are disrupting normal respiration, artificial ventilation should begin immediately if the athlete's respiration is ineffective or nonexistent. Insufficient respiration, or hypoventilation, is observed when the breathing rate is below 10 breaths per minute or above 30 breaths per minutes, indicating inadequate rate or volume, respectively. Insufficient respiration requires immediate care from the sports emergency care team in order to support central nervous and cardiovascular systems functions. Decreased respiration rates are associated with the onset of cardiac complications that will intensify a critical situation.[21,22] In addition, the spinal cord may suffer a 20% to 30% decline in oxygenation due to swelling and vascular compromise following injury.[16] The combined effect of declining oxygenation due to injury and decreased plasma oxygen concentrations resulting from insufficient respiration can significantly magnify the ischemic condition experienced by the spinal cord following injury.

If the athlete is breathing adequately, there is no immediate need to use manual or mechanical procedures to ensure that he or she is receiving ample oxygen.[22,23] However, if respiratory irregularities exist, the sports emergency care team must be prepared to render care. Rendering care to an athlete with a potential CSI in protective athletic equipment may require the sports emergency care team to extract the facemask from a protective athletic football helmet. Unlike motorcycle helmets, a properly fitted football helmet can aid the sports emergency care team in maintaining immobilization of the head and neck during transfer and transport, thereby protecting the cervical spine from further injury. Additionally, extraction of the facemask from a football helmet is preferred to complete helmet removal because it is associated with significantly less extraneous movement of the head and neck. Therefore, leaving a football helmet in place while extracting the facemask to gain access to an athlete with a potential CSI reduces the risk of secondary injury.[24]

The considerable attention given to facemask extraction throughout the years is a testament to the necessity of possessing the psychomotor skills required to efficiently remove a facemask.[22,25-29] However, few sports health care professionals have an appreciation as to how difficult it is to remove a facemask. The sports emergency care team must undertake regular rehearsal to ensure that each member possesses the psychomotor skills required to efficiently extract a facemask from an athletic helmet in an emergency. The effective sports emergency care team is able to accomplish this task in 30 seconds to 60 seconds. When facemask extraction is required, complete extraction of the facemask from the helmet is preferred to retraction of the facemask. Complete extraction of the facemask results in less extraneous cervical spine movement compared to facemask retraction, while a retracted facemask could provide a lever through which torque could be applied to the cervical spine during the care and management process.[26] Additionally, there seems to be little time-saving benefit to retraction relative to extraction of a facemask since retraction of the facemask requires releasing the more difficult lateral facemask fasteners from the football helmet while leaving the relatively easy-to-release forehead fasteners in place. If there is any time savings of retraction versus extraction of a facemask, it is likely minimal and is offset by the movement that would be applied to the injured cervical spine if contact were to be made with the retracted facemask while the sports emergency care team rendered care.

The equipment used to extract a facemask is a team decision. Advantages and disadvantages of all facemask extraction equipment must be carefully considered. The effectiveness of any facemask extraction tool is a product of the time required for extraction and the movement within the cervical spine during extraction.[25,26,28] There are various facemask fasteners used to secure facemasks to athletic helmets. A facemask removal tool must be evaluated by the sports emergency care team based on time and motions relative to all the various fasteners in use. Efficient sports emergency care teams are likely to find a combined tool approach (ie, a cutting tool such as the FMxtractor and a power screwdriver) most beneficial.[30] Facemask removal techniques for the various facemask fasteners in use will be discussed later in the chapter.

Circulation

Once management for breathing has been rendered, the sports emergency care team will check circulation. Normal physiological function of the cardiovascular system ensures adequate blood flow throughout the body. This requires that the heart functions properly, an adequate amount of blood circulates in the body, and that blood vessels are capable of properly adjusting blood flow. Disruption of neurological tissues may interrupt communications between the brainstem and sympathetic neurons. The result is failure of the cardiovascular system to maintain adequate blood flow throughout the body, resulting in systemic vasodilatation and decreased cardiac function leading to vasomotor shock, postural hypotension, and edema in the lower extremities.[31] Other complications due to failure of the cardiovascular system include bradycardia, decreased myocardial contractility, hypothermia, and a predisposition to supraventricular tachycardia (SVT). Cardiac complications relating to neural damage typically arise due to 2 possible scenarios. One possible scenario involves immediate cardiac arrest resulting from damage at the C1 level. Management of immediate cardiac arrest would necessarily supersede specific care of the cervical spine. A second scenario involves injury to the cervical spine above the C4 level that affects the phrenic nerve, resulting in immediate or delayed decreased respiratory efforts due to loss of function of the diaphragm. If cardiac arrest is immediate, management of the cardiac arrest, again, supersedes care for a CSI. However, if the effects on the cardiovascular system are delayed, the sports emergency care team has an opportunity to assess and prepare for the possible onset of cardiac complications, possibly avoiding the onset altogether.[13]

Cardiovascular function can be readily assessed by the sports emergency care team through conscientious monitoring of the injured athlete's pulse and respiration, which provide clues as to the status of blood pressure and the overall status of the cardiovascular system. Normal resting pulse rate for adults ranges from 60 beats per minute to 100 beats per minute. It should be noted that a trained athlete might have a significantly lower resting heart rate. Conversely, an athlete participating in physical activity may have a higher-than-normal heart rate that should begin to normalize shortly after cessation of activity. The presence of a strong, rapid pulse is to be expected in athletes during competition. A better indicator of problems related to pulse and blood pressure is a delay in normalization. Normal systolic blood pressure for a 15-year-old to 20-year old male is 115 mm Hg to 120 mm Hg. Normal diastolic pressure ranges from 75 mm Hg to 80 mm Hg. The average pressure for a female in the same age range is generally 8 mm Hg to 10 mm Hg lower than that of males.

In general, determination of a carotid pulse indicates a systolic pressure above 60 mm Hg. The presence of the femoral pulse indicates a systolic pressure of between 70 mm Hg and 80 mm Hg. If the radial pulse is present, the systolic pressure is at least above 90 mm Hg, indicating a minimal blood pressure is present. A conscientious check of the athlete's nail beds and extremity temperature can also be used to grossly assess tissue perfusion, possibly indicating cardiovascular system failure. Although absence of the carotid pulse determines the need for CPR or defibrillation, a weak or absent radial pulse, bradycardia, or perfusion abnormalities are significant indicators of hypotension and oncoming cardiac complications due to failure of the cardiovascular system.[22]

A radial pulse check provides the sports emergency care team with an immediate initial assessment of cardiovascular function that is vital to making primary assessment and care decisions for the spine-injured athlete. Hypotension leads to decreased cord perfusion and consequent worsening of deficit.[20] If proper cardiovascular function is not maintained, hypotension may facilitate the progression of spinal shock. As a result of decreased oxygen delivery to the neural tissues, even a complete lesion may be worsened by allowing associated necrosis to progress throughout the neural tissues.

When assessing and monitoring an athlete's vital signs, it is important that the sports emergency care team realize that the measures discussed here are for the normal person at rest. Athletes' vital signs may vary from norms due to such factors as cardiovascular conditioning, body size, and physical exertion. Cardiovascular conditioning, body size, and exertion are factors that must be taken into account when determining if any variations from vital sign norms actually indicate bradycardia, hypoventilation, or cardiac complication that requires immediate care.

SEVERE BLEEDING, SHOCK, AND SPINAL INJURY

In completing the ABC Sx3 primary assessment, the sports emergency care team should quickly assess the athlete for and control any major bleeding. Assessing and treating for shock should also be considered. Temperature is an important consideration in treating any injured athlete for shock. Internal temperature regulation is dependent upon interrelations between the hypothalamus, autonomic nervous system (ANS), and the cardiovascular system. Disruption of the ANS affects the body's ability to react to changes in temperature through vasodilatation and vasoconstriction. The sweating mechanism may become disrupted, leading it to react to stresses other than increasing temperature (ie, autonomic hyperreflexia).[32] The body assumes the temperature of the surroundings (poikilothermia) when there is severe CSI due to the diminished ability to react to increasing body temperature. Therefore, it is vital to avoid and render treatment for extreme temperatures. Characteristically, low body temperature presents with chills, chattering teeth, blue lips, goose bumps, and/or pale skin.[22]

Spinal injury is the focus of this chapter. A simple gross motor and sensory test to determine any loss of strength or sensation should be used. Though upper and lower neurological screens are effective means of determining the lesion site and involved neural tissue, this information is quite often much more than is needed to determine the immediate course of care. The most important aspect of this stage of care is the informed decision to transport and to ensure that no further injury results from the process. There are many signs and symptoms that are indicative of the need for conservative measures that will be greater influences on the decision to immobilize and transfer the athlete than the neurological screen. Unconsciousness and other general signs and symptoms may indicate the need for immobilization and transfer prior to the more involved neurological screening. Still, the sports health care professional must possess the upper and lower neurological screen assessment skills in order to safely rule out neurological involvement during potential CSI situations that are not immediately recognizable.

Other injuries such as burners and stingers present with similar neurological presentations. The sports health care professional must be able to distinguish between other injuries involving neurological presentations. If spinal cord injury cannot be definitively ruled out, the athlete must be immobilized and transported. Some of the distinguishing characteristics that can help determine whether an injury involves the cervical spine will be discussed later.

THE "RULE OF 100"

As previously stated, a conscientious primary assessment of an athlete with a possible spinal injury can yield vital clues that may indicate the presence of significant injury in the absence of the more obvious gross neurological signs and symptoms most often associated with a spinal injury. An effective means of analyzing the information gathered during the acute primary injury assessment with regard to spinal shock is comparing the initial measure to the "Rule of 100" associated with vital signs trending.

Action may be warranted when any of these initial measures fall outside of the "Rule of 100." The "Rule of 100" can be very helpful in ruling out possible cardiopulmonary conditions that can be subtle indicators of the underlying presence of spinal shock. According to the "Rule of 100," if the pulse or temperature is less than 100 or the systolic blood pressure is greater than 100, significant injury is less likely, assuming there are no other indicators of significant injury.

Possible spinal injury will become evident early in the primary assessment, as will any need for CPR or defibrillation. Care for the spinal cord during administration of CPR and/or cardiac defibrillation is not the primary objective in light of respiratory or cardiac emergencies. However, sports emergency care team members must possess the skills necessary to protect the spine from further injury while caring for immediate medical emergencies. In athletics, caring for immediate life-threatening injuries in addition to spinal injuries may involve management of protective athletic equipment, including protective shoulder pads, athletic helmets, and facemasks.

With proper preparation, most immediate life-threatening conditions identified during the primary assessment can be managed with little interference from protective athletic equipment. It has been demonstrated that proper airway evaluation, establishment, maintenance, and rescue breathing can be administered by removing the facemask from protective athletic helmets, while leaving the helmet and shoulder pads in place.[18,24,33,34] Cutting away the athlete's jersey, shoulder pad strings, and any underclothing is sufficient for effective cardiac monitoring as long as the skin is dry.[22] It has also been demonstrated that CPR can be effectively administered with the shoulder pads in place by spreading the pads wide enough apart to expose the chest.[33,35] Incorporation of these techniques allows the majority of emergent situations to be effectively cared for while leaving the athlete's equipment in place, thus protecting the spine from further injury due to excessive and unnecessary movement. All sports emergency care team members should possess the skills to effectively perform the techniques required for effective equipment management.

Complete equipment removal in order to expose the athlete for further assessment is unnecessary in caring for the spine-injured athlete. If the athlete complains of chest pain or shortness of breath, the chest must be exposed to allow for evaluation of lung sounds and cardiac monitoring. These evaluations can be accomplished without complete removal of the equipment. When exposing large portions of the body, steps must be taken to protect the athlete from hypothermia. This is especially true in cases of spinal cord injury when the body's thermoregulatory systems may be impaired.

As outlined previously, exposure of the chest can be accomplished by cutting away the jersey, the strings and straps securing the pads in place, and any clothing worn under the pads. The shoulder pads can then be carefully spread apart to allow further evaluation. When spreading the shoulder pads, be aware of the system used to secure the pads posteriorly. In some systems, spreading the anterior plates of more rigid pads may cause the straps or plates to bunch together, resulting in discomfort or undesired movement.

Progressive Algorithm for the Management of the Spine-Injured Athlete

Completion of the primary survey may provide vital information that indicates the need for immediate life-saving techniques or the need for immediate immobilization and transport of the athlete to a regional spinal trauma center. However, obvious signs and symptoms of life-threatening cervical spine trauma may not be immediately apparent. If the primary survey does not indicate the need for immediate transport to a regional spine injury trauma center, the effective sports emergency care team is prepared to conduct a thorough secondary survey that involves a progression of careful steps to determine if more subtle signs and symptoms are present.

The Progressive Algorithm for the Management of the Spine-Injured Athlete (PA) approach is used to assess for more subtle signs and symptoms of CSI for 4 specific and important conditions (Figure 6-3). First, the PA approach allows the sports emergency care team to develop an on-field assessment strategy that is organized and logical. With the organized and logical assessment PA strategy, the sports emergency care team is less likely to forget to assess some particular sign or symptom. Second, the organized PA approach allows the sports emergency care team to build in failsafe "fuses," or indicators that immediate transport of the athlete to a regional trauma center is required. The PA presented here is a progressive evaluation that permits more movement as the sports emergency care team becomes more confident that a CSI does not exist. There is a failsafe fuse at each progressive step in this evaluation. If certain signs and symptoms are observed during any particular stage of the assessment, the fuse is blown and the sports emergency care team activates EMS to aid in caring for and transporting the athlete. Once a fuse is blown in the PA and EMS is activated, the team's CSI assessment for the purpose of determining the need to transporting the athlete is over. The initial caregivers maintain vital signs while waiting for EMS team members to arrive. Together, the sports emergency care team conducts necessary ongoing assessment during

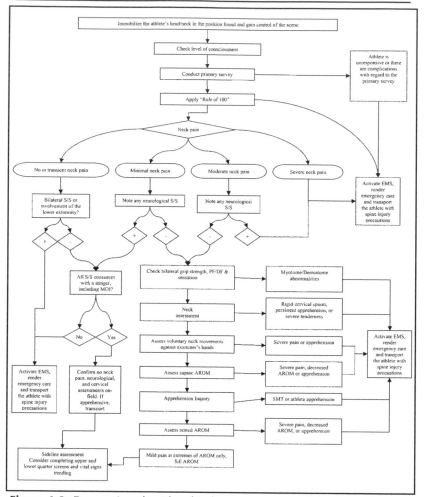

Figure 6-3. Progressive algorithm for the management of the cervical spine-injured athlete. (© Sports Medicine Concepts. Reproduced with permission.)

transfer of the athlete to a rigid support, immobilization, and transport of the athlete to a regional spinal trauma center. After the PA indicates the need for transport, unnecessary assessment should be avoided because it increases the likelihood of extraneous movement of the athlete and provides an opportunity for apparent improvements in signs and symptoms to cause the sports emergency care team to mistakenly reverse a decision to transport.

The third reason for the PA approach is that the PA allows the sports emergency care team to quickly differentiate between injuries to the cervical spine and other injuries that present with similar signs and symptoms. In the example provided here, signs and symptoms closely associated with burners, stingers, and soft tissue injuries are built in. Generally, the difference between CSI and other soft tissue injuries involves the location of the signs and symptoms and the mechanism of injury. The sports emergency care team must be very suspicious of pain or point tenderness along the vertebral column. If pain or point tenderness along the vertebral column is combined with an axial load mechanism, a CSI must be assumed. Athletes who have suffered some other cervical soft tissue injury will likely present with pain and point tenderness in the upper trapezius muscle, the sternocleidomastoid muscle, or otherwise off midline of the cervical vertebral column. Athletes suspected of having suffered a burner or stinger must present with the specific pattern of signs and symptoms that historically have defined a burner. This includes a mechanism of injury of lateral bending of the neck and depression of the ipsilateral shoulder with radicular signs and symptoms isolated in the ipsilateral upper extremity. If there is any deviation from these historical presentations, a CSI must be assumed.

Finally, the PA approach is suggested because the acquisition of vital information is necessary to progress from one stage to the next in the PA. Every step in the PA requires the acquisition of certain vital information in order to decide if the athlete needs to be transported or if the sports emergency care team can continue to the next stage of the assessment. If the information required to make the decision to transport or to continue with the assessment cannot be acquired because the athlete is in an altered state of consciousness or is otherwise not able to verbalize answers to specific questions, then serious injury to the cervical spine or head must be assumed and the decision to transport the athlete must be made.

Transfer and Immobilization

When a fuse is blown during the PA, EMS must be activated and the sports emergency care team must begin preparing the athlete for transport to a regional trauma center. This process is initiated with the transfer of the athlete to a rigid immobilization support. For the athlete in protective football equipment, the combination of football shoulder pads and helmet serve the athlete and the sports emergency care team well in maintaining immobilization and axial alignment during transfer to a rigid immobilization system. Therefore, it is suggested that this equipment be left in place whenever possible.[24,36]

Transfer of the spine-injured athlete is a technique that has received much attention. The most common technique for repositioning of the athlete is the log-roll.[37] However, the flat-lift, lift-slide maneuver, and 6-person lift have also been shown to be an effective means of transferring an injured athlete to a rigid support.[38] When using the log-roll maneuver, the team must pay

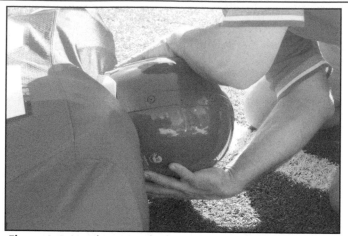

Figure 6-4. Hand position for log-roll maneuver.

particular attention to lumbar and thoracic as well as cervical movements that have been associated with this technique. This is especially true in the presence of protective sporting equipment. The team member responsible for stabilization of the head and neck during the log-roll maneuver can help ensure a smooth transition of the head and neck from the prone position to the supine by reversing his or her hands on the athlete's helmet prior to rolling the athlete (Figure 6-4). Also, if this individual assumes a position at the head of the immobilization device (where the athlete will end up when the log-roll is completed) while reaching with his or her arms and hands to stabilize (much like the position a baseball catcher uses to reach for a low and outside pitch), a much smoother transition will ensue. Prior to the log-roll, be sure the team is positioned such that the athlete is not log-rolled over the facemask (Figure 6-5). Log-rolling over the facemask will force the neck into extension.

During a log-roll, the sports emergency care team must be conscious of, and prepared to manage, a 1-inch to 2-inch space between the back of an athlete's head or helmet and the ground or rigid immobilization device following log-rolling an athlete to the supine position, even when both the helmet and shoulder pads have been left in place. Failure to anticipate and account for the gap between the back of the athlete's head and the ground or rigid support will result in dangerous extension of the neck.[39] A simple solution is to pack and fill all voids using towels that can be folded and placed under the head or helmet as the athlete is log-rolled (Figure 6-6). Certain commercial rigid support devices that are equipped with padding may also be evaluated for use by the sports emergency care team. Traditional backboards have been widely used to immobilize potential spinal cord injuries without much change since the 1960s. When combined with immobilization devices, including straps,

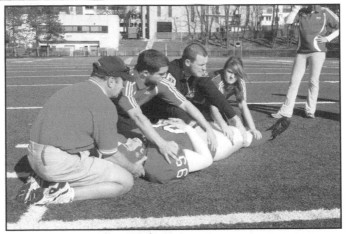

Figure 6-5. Log-roll procedure.

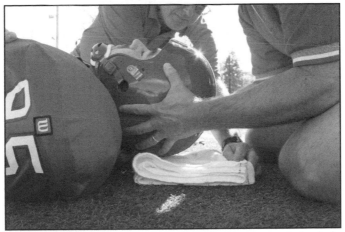

Figure 6-6. A towel can be used to fill the gap beneath the helmet and the ground.

cervical collars, and head immobilization devices, the backboard is the standard rigid immobilization device used today.[35,37,40,41]

The 6-plus-person lift is another method of transferring an injured athlete to a spine board.[24] During the 6-plus-person lift (Figure 6-7), one team member maintains manual, inline stabilization of the head, while team members on both sides of the athlete lift at the athlete's upper torso, hips and pelvis, and legs. Team members responsible for lifting the upper torso place one hand underneath the shoulder and another underneath the torso just above the pelvis. Team members responsible for lifting the hip and pelvis place one hand

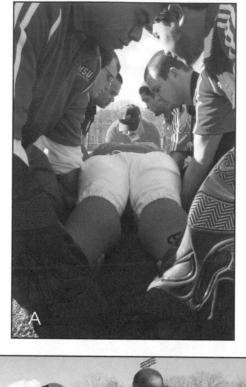

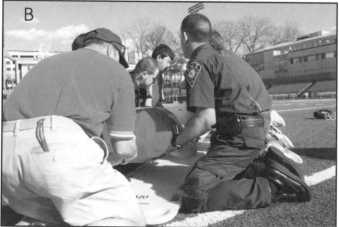

Figure 6-7. 6-plus-person technique.

beneath the victim's lower torso, and another beneath the thigh. Team members lifting the legs place hands beneath the legs above and below the knees. The team member responsible for supporting the head directs the other team members to raise the injured athlete off the ground, instructs another rescuer to slide the board beneath the athlete, then instructs the team members to gently lower the athlete onto the spine board. Another variation of the 6-plus-person lift is called the lift-slide technique. The same lift is performed with one team member at the head, one team member straddling and lifting the chest/torso, one team member straddling and lifting the hips and pelvis, and one team member straddling and lifting the legs. Once the athlete is lifted, a fifth team member slides the spine board beneath the athlete.

The log-roll, lift-slide, and 6-plus-person lift can be effective methods of transferring a spine-injured athlete to a rigid support device. The sports emergency care team should evaluate these techniques for adoption into its protocol for transferring an athlete with a potential CSI to a rigid support. Regardless of the method employed, the sports emergency care team must make a conscious decision to rehearse transfer techniques regularly to ensure that the technique employed minimizes the chance for unwanted movement of the athlete. When reviewing the log-roll and lift-slide methods for transferring an injured athlete, the sports emergency care team must also consider the rigid support to which the athlete will be transferred. Regular-sized backboards may be too small for larger athletes. Oversized backboards, or sports boards, may be more appropriate for larger athletes but may not fit in all ambulances and are too large for most medical evacuation helicopters (Figure 6-8).

Once the athlete is transferred to a rigid support device, stabilization of the head and neck is accomplished via the application of appropriate cervical immobilization devices and, in some instances, continued manual stabilization (Figure 6-9). Application of a cervical collar is not required when immobilizing an athlete in football shoulder pads and a protective helmet. In fact, the use of cervical immobilization collars may be contraindicated all together during immobilization of the injured football or hockey player. Since cervical immobilization collars are not designed for use with protective athletic equipment, the application of these collars results in significant and unnecessary movement of adjacent cervical vertebrae.[42]

Two precautionary measures should be taken prior to transferring and securing the athlete to a rigid immobilization device in order to further reduce the risk of unnecessary movement. First, regardless of the athlete's present condition, the facemask should be removed from the athlete's helmet upon determining the need to transport the athlete and prior to transferring the athlete to a rigid support. Second, the shoulder pads should be prepared after the athlete has been transferred. Shoulder pads are prepared by first cutting the athlete's jersey to expose the shoulder pads. Next, the shoulder pad's lateral elastic straps followed by the breast plate laces and any

Figure 6-8. Backboards are available in different sizes.

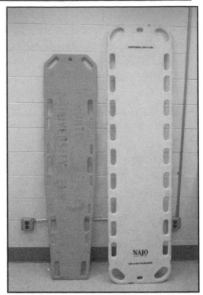

Figure 6-9. Use of a cervical immobilization device.

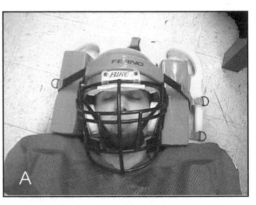

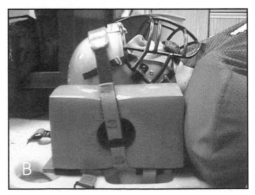

undergarments should be cut. Cutting the elastic straps prior to cutting the breast plate strings may reduce unwanted movement caused by the elastic straps pulling the breast plate apart when strings holding the breast plate together are cut. These measures will facilitate any emergency procedures that might be required should the athlete's condition worsen during transport by providing EMS with adequate access to the athlete without the movement and time associated with complete equipment removal.

Facemask Removal

Removal of the athlete's facemask as a precautionary measure prior to transport significantly eases the work of EMS should a breathing emergency arise during transport by providing immediate airway access while avoiding the time delays and extraneous movement that would result from either facemask or helmet removal during transport. With continued practice and rehearsal, the facemask of any helmet can quickly and safely be removed with minimal risk of extraneous movement of the cervical spine. Thus, it is suggested that the facemask be removed as a precautionary measure in every potential CSI.

Today there are 4 different facemask fasteners that are used to secure facemasks to football helmets, including the standard loop strap, Shockblocker (Riddell, Elyria, Ohio), Stabilizer (Innovative Athletic Products, Strongsville, Ohio), and Revolution (Riddell, Elyria, Ohio). The various facemask fasteners presently in use are all widely available and all but the Revolution are easily retrofitted to any football helmet. Sports emergency care professionals responsible for the care of critically injured football players must be prepared to efficiently remove each of these facemask fasteners during care for a critically injured athlete. Although the fasteners that secure facemasks to lacrosse, hockey, and softball helmets may be similar to those securing facemasks to football helmets, the strength of the argument for facemask removal rather than protective helmet removal has yet to be determined for these protective athletic helmets. Historically, sports emergency care professionals have relied on power screwdrivers and cutting tools, such as the FMxtractor, anvil pruner, Trainers' Angel, and modified PVC pipe cutter to remove the loop strap fasteners securing facemasks to protective athletic helmets (Figure 6-10). The following section details specific techniques that sports emergency care team members may consider when evaluating different cutting tools and practicing facemask removal procedure.[43] It is difficult to fully demonstrate the various techniques used to cut through various facemask fasteners within the confines of a textbook. Therefore, it is strongly suggested that sports emergency care personnel acquire proper hands-on training in emergency facemask removal for a more thorough review of facemask removal techniques.

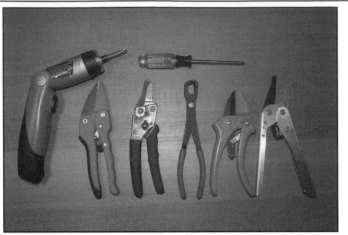

Figure 6-10. Facemask removal tools.

LOOP STRAP FASTENERS

The forehead fasteners of every football helmet are similar, using a standard loop strap fastener consisting of a fixed screw end and a loop portion (Figure 6-11). The Revolution helmet uses slightly smaller versions of the standard loop strap fastener to secure the facemask to the forehead of the helmet. To release the forehead loop strap fasteners, position the cutting blade and opposing buttress of the cutting tool as depicted in Figure 6-12A. This will result in the fixed screw portion of the loop strap to remain fixed to the helmet shell while the loop portion of the fastener remains on the facemask bar (Figure 6-12B). If the ends of the cutting device are not resting firmly against the helmet shell, the bottom portion of the loop strap is not likely to be completely transected, resulting in the inability to release the facemask bar from the loop strap.

Another option for cutting the loop strap that may be advantageous when grip strength is an issue is to complete an initial cut as described above but cut through only the top portion of the loop strap. Then position the buttress of the cutting tool to make a second cut as depicted in Figure 6-13. This technique will release an area of plastic from the loop strap fastener sufficient to allow the facemask bar to be removed (Figure 6-14).

Loop strap fasteners along the sides of the football helmet pose a significant challenge to emergent facemask removal. To facilitate removal of loop strap fasteners along the sides of the helmet, first observe how the loop strap is positioned relative to the facemask bars. If there is enough clearance between the adjacent facemask bars and the loop strap, place the cutting tool over the loop strap fastener (Figure 6-15). If the approach

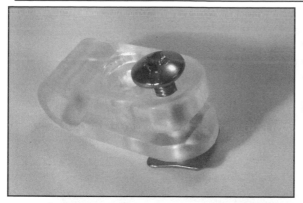

Figure 6-11. Standard loop strap facemask fastener with screw and t-nut. (© Sports Medicine Concepts. Reproduced with permission.)

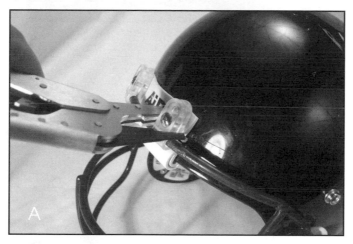

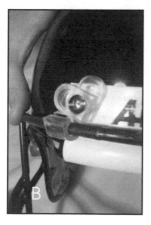

Figure 6-12. Technique for cutting standard forehead facemask fasteners results in the fastener being completely transected at its midsection. (© Sports Medicine Concepts. Reproduced with permission.)

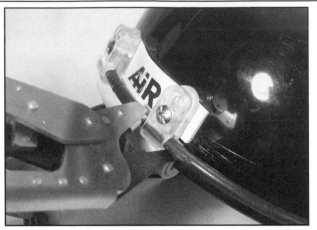

Figure 6-13. Second technique for cutting forehead standard loop strap facemask fasteners may require less grip strength to complete. (© Sports Medicine Concepts. Reproduced with permission.)

Figure 6-14. Standard side loop strap facemask fasteners after being cut using alternate method. (© Sports Medicine Concepts. Reproduced with permission.)

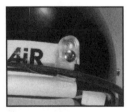

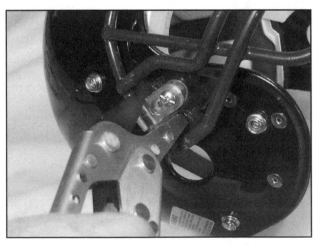

Figure 6-15. Technique for cutting standard loop strap facemask fasteners on the sides of football helmets. (© Sports Medicine Concepts. Reproduced with permission.)

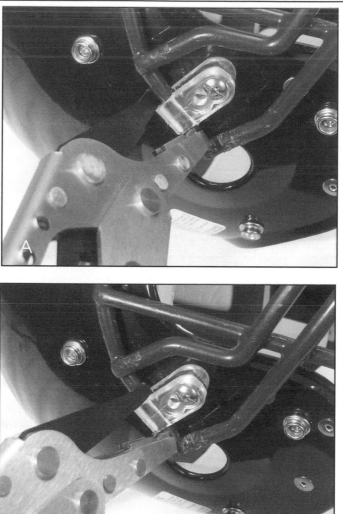

Figure 6-16. Second technique for cutting standard loop strap facemask fasteners on the sides of football helmets. (© Sports Medicine Concepts. Reproduced with permission.)

detailed in Figure 6-15 does not successfully release the facemask bar from the loop strap after the first attempt, try repositioning the cutting device by placing the buttress of the cutting tool on the facemask bar as depicted in Figure 6-16. The result will be a gap in the loop strap that is wide enough for the facemask bar to be pulled through.

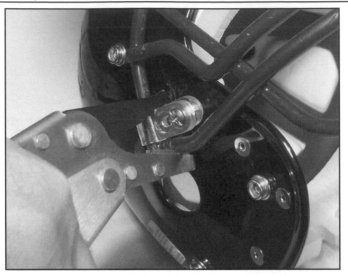

Figure 6-17. A third technique for cutting standard side loop strap fasteners on football helmets. (© Sports Medicine Concepts. Reproduced with permission.)

If there is not ample room to position the cutting tool over the loop strap fastener within the confines of the adjacent facemask bars, place the buttress of the cutting tool on the facemask bar at one side of the loop strap with the cutting blade positioned at the opposite side as depicted in Figure 6-16. Approximate the ends of the cutting tool to cut through the top half of the loop strap. Finally, leaving the buttress on the facemask bar, reposition the cutting blade parallel to the opposite side of the facemask bar and, again, cut the top half of the loop strap (see Figure 6-16). The result will be a gap in the loop strap that is wide enough for the facemask bar to be pulled through.

If the loop strap fastener is positioned off-center relative to the adjacent facemask bars, it may be possible to rest the buttress of the cutting tool on the outside edge of the facemask bar with the cutting blade extended across the width of the loop strap fastener and resting firmly on the helmet shell (Figure 6-17). While in this position, approximate the ends of the cutting tool to transect the fastener at its midpoint. Often this technique results in a small remnant of plastic remaining uncut. To avoid the plastic remnant, end this cut by slightly rotating the approximated handles of the cutting tool around the facemask bar to allow the cutting blade to completely cut the loop strap. If the entire depth of the loop strap fastener is not completely transected, try repositioning as depicted in Figure 6-16.

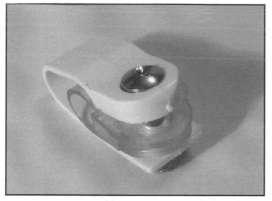

Figure 6-18. Shock-blocker facemask fastener with screw and t-nut. (© Sports Medicine Concepts. Reproduced with permission.)

The same cutting options described for cutting standard loop strap fasteners can be applied to the other fastener variations. However, there are some considerations that can facilitate cutting these fasteners.

Shockblocker

The Shockblocker is designed with a hard outer plastic loop and a more pliable inner loop (Figure 6-18). The outer loop provides rigid support while the inner loop may provide some protection from concussion injury by absorbing some of the force from a blow to the facemask.

Cut the Shockblocker by placing the buttress and cutting blade over the fastener such that the top half of both the inner and outer loops can be cut simultaneously using one of the techniques outlined previously. Then simply push the inner and outer layer out of the way and pull the facemask bar out from the fastener (Figure 6-19).

Stabilizer

The Stabilizer fasteners come in thick and thin modes. Thick or thin fasteners are used depending on the circumference of the facemask bar being fixed to the football helmet shell. Stabilizer fasteners are also specifically designed for the right and left sides of the helmet. The Stabilizer fastener has a thin secondary plastic loop strap that may provide additional support and may help prevent concussion injury by absorbing some of the force from a blow to the facemask. Look for the depression near the front of the loop portion of the fastener (Figure 6-20). This area of the Stabilizer has the least amount of plastic and may provide the least amount of resistance to cutting.

Begin cutting the Stabilizer fastener by first cutting the fastener's secondary loop strap (Figure 6-21). It is much more difficult to cut the secondary loop strap after the main body of the fastener has been cut. After cutting through the secondary loop strap, the main body of the Stabilizer can be cut by placing

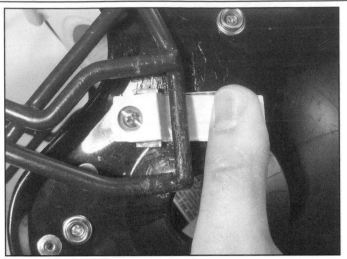

Figure 6-19. The Shockblocker may only require a single cut through both its inner and outer loop. (© Sports Medicine Concepts. Reproduced with permission.)

Figure 6-20. Position the cutting tool at the depression in the Stabilizer facemask fasteners. (© Sports Medicine Concepts. Reproduced with permission.)

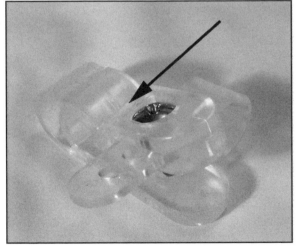

the buttress and blade of the cutting tool on either side of the fastener (Figures 6-22 through 6-24).

Revolution

The Revolution fastener is presently manufactured with 2 access slots to facilitate cutting the fastener. When the fastener is properly mounted

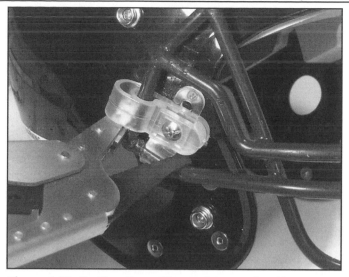

Figure 6-21. Position the cutting tool to cut the thin support loop before cutting the main body of the Stabilizer. (© Sports Medicine Concepts. Reproduced with permission.)

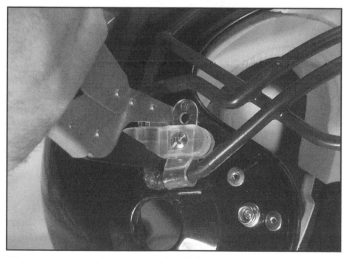

Figure 6-22. Cut the main body of the Stabilizer at the depression between the loop portion and fixed screw end. (© Sports Medicine Concepts. Reproduced with permission.)

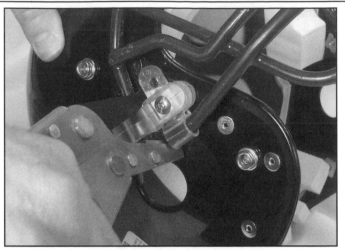

Figure 6-23. Alternate tool position to cut Stabilizer facemask fastener. (© Sports Medicine Concepts. Reproduced with permission.)

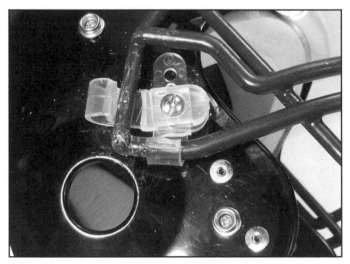

Figure 6-24. Stabilizer facemask fastener after using a 3-cut approach. This approach may require the least amount of grip strength to complete. (© Sports Medicine Concepts. Reproduced with permission.)

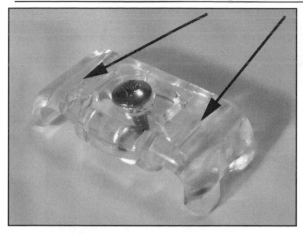

Figure 6-25. Access slots for cutting the Revolution facemask fastener. (© Sports Medicine Concepts. Reproduced with permission.)

on the helmet, the fore access slot is milled at approximately 12 degrees to 15 degrees while the aft access slot is milled perpendicular to the helmet shell (Figure 6-25). According to Revolution manufacturer recommendations, the fore access slot should be cut first, followed by the aft. If your team is presently outfitted with Revolution helmets, be sure to check all helmets to ensure that the fasteners have access slots. Without access slots, facemask removal is limited to unscrewing the fastener hardware. If you find fasteners without access slots, replace the fasteners with those that do have access slots immediately.

Many have come to prefer the screwdriver as the first option for removing the Revolution fastener (Figure 6-26). The screwdriver has been found to be a viable first option. However, due to the potential for hardware failure, a back-up cutting option is recommended.[30]

The Revolution manufacturer has specific instructions for cutting the Revolution fastener. These instructions must be followed precisely for the most effective and timely release of the fastener. To release the Revolution fastener, identify the fore access slot. Allow the cutting blade of the tool to fall into the access slot at 12 degrees to 15 degrees, coming to rest on the helmet shell. Then, position the buttress of the cutting tool on the outside of the facemask bar (Figure 6-27). Approximate the ends of the cutting tool and ease the blade through the fastener. Reverse the position of the cutting tool and repeat the process to cut through the remaining portion of the fastener using the fore access slot (Figure 6-28). Next, repeat the process using the aft access slot. Keep in mind that the aft access slots are cut perpendicular to the helmet shell; therefore, the blade of the cutting tool should be directed straight into the access slot, not at a 12-degree to 15-degree angle. When initiating the cut, be sure that the blade rests firmly against the helmet shell. Rotate the handles of the cutting tool slightly forward after the blade contacts the facemask bar to

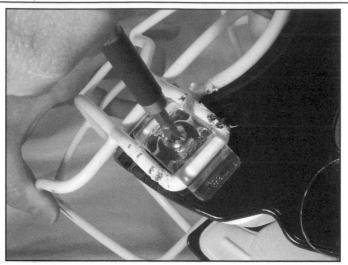

Figure 6-26. Using a screwdriver to release the Revolution face-mask fastener. (© Sports Medicine Concepts. Reproduced with permission.)

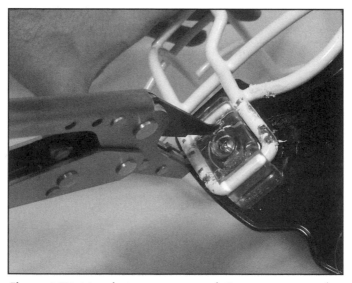

Figure 6-27. Manufacturer recommendations state to cut the fore access slots of the Revolution fastener first. (© Sports Medicine Concepts. Reproduced with permission.)

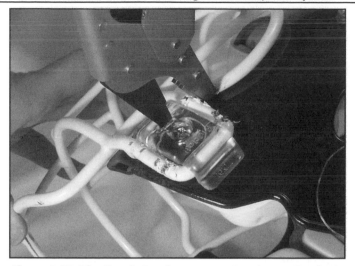

Figure 6-28. The Revolution fastener requires 4 cuts, 2 at both the fore and aft access slots. (© Sports Medicine Concepts. Reproduced with permission.)

complete the cut. When the Revolution fastener is properly fixed to the helmet and the cutting tool makes an efficient cut, each end of the Revolution fastener will fall away, exposing the facemask bars (Figure 6-29). If the Revolution fastener remains in position after cutting, reposition the cutting tool to ensure that the fastener has been completely transected. In some cases, the Revolution fastener will remain in place even after completely transecting both ends. This is due to the pressure that is applied to the fastener. If this happens, simply ease the fastener off of the facemask bar. If this fails, use a screwdriver to unscrew the fastener from the helmet.

Initial Emergency Room Trauma Assessment

Once the facemask has been removed and the shoulder pads properly prepared prior to transporting an athlete with a potential CSI, there is little chance that the helmet and shoulder pads will have to be removed from the athlete until after an initial ER trauma assessment has been completed.

In the absence of life-threatening conditions, initial ER assessment begins with the initial radiographic plain film trauma evaluation performed prior to removal of any equipment from the athlete. The initial ER radiographic film trauma series typically involves horizontal cross-table lateral (HL), anteroposterior (AP), oblique, and pillar films. Though HL films alone are not

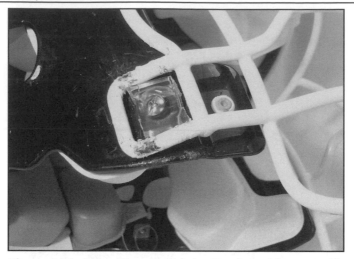

Figure 6-29. The midsection of the Revolution fastener will remain fixed to the helmet, but will permit the facemask to be lifted off the helmet. (© Sports Medicine Concepts. Reproduced with permission.)

conclusive, they are generally sufficient to rule out gross instability in the cervical spine. Initial HL radiographic films provide the ER personnel with a general understanding of the osseous condition of the cervical vertebrae. The information provided on the HL views can be used by ER personnel in preparation for removing all protective equipment from the athlete in order to conduct a more thorough radiographic assessment. All protective equipment should be removed from the athlete using the spine injury precautions detailed below, regardless of what is depicted on the HL radiographic films.

Once protective equipment has been removed from the athlete, more extensive radiographic evaluation, including AP and additional HL views, using plain film are taken to further evaluate bony instability. Routine AP views are used to evaluate the integrity and alignment of the superior and inferior vertebral end plates, pedicles, and spinous processes of C3–C7. An open-mouth AP view is necessary for evaluation of C1–C2. The open-mouth AP is completed in order to observe that the odontoid process is equidistant from the lateral masses of C1, that C1 and C2 lateral masses are aligned, and the presence of a mach effect (ie, a simulated fracture caused by C1 projecting over the dens). The additional HL views following protective equipment removal allow observation of the soft tissues, lordotic curve, disk space, posterior cortical margins of articular processes, spinolaminar lines, facets, intervertebral height, and interspinous distances of the spinous processes. Occasionally, C6–C7 and the odontoid process are obscured in the HL view by the shoulder girdle and mandible respectively. If C6–C7 and the odontoid process are obscured, the swimmer's position may be used. To complete the initial radiographic plain film series, oblique and pillar views are completed to assess the interfacetal joints, laminae, intervertebral foramen, and lateral masses. If the athlete is unconscious or unstable, the complete radiographic plain film series may be contraindicated. If the complete initial radiographic plain film assessment is contraindicated, computerized tomography (CT) may used to complete the initial trauma assessment. When indicated, CT and fluoroscopy are used for more extensive evaluation of the vertebrae and canal, while myelonography may be combined with CT or magnetic resonance imaging (MRI) for evaluation of spinal cord and nerve root damage. Generally, fluoroscopy and CT are useful for specific views under direct control. CT is useful when vertebrae are superimposed or when it is necessary to observe a specific vertebral component, especially in evaluating the pedicle, lamina, cord, and canal.

Specific evaluation of the spinal cord and nerve roots requires myelography, CT, and/or MRI combined with contrast enhancement. Myelogram combined with a subarachnoid injection of contrast agent is used for observation of the subarachnoid space, cord, and nerve roots. MRI and CT following myelogram allows specific observation of the cord and canal contents.

Recent advances in CT and MRI have had important implications in the evaluation of alignment and integrity of bony structures, ligamentous stability, extradural mass effects resulting from osteophytes, herniated disks, fracture fragments and hematomas, and spinal cord status. MRI has been reported to be superior to CT for visualizing extradural mass effects and cord injury because of its sensitivity to subtle abnormalities, including syringomyelia. CT is unable to detect small areas of edema and swelling; therefore, only gross compression or altered cord contour is observable using CT. MRI has also been found to be more beneficial for analysis of discs because it is noninvasive and multiplanar. However, MRI is limited in detecting fractures and dislocations unless there is gross displacement and cord impingement. Generally, MRI is the modality of choice for soft tissue evaluation.[44]

Conversely, CT is especially sensitive to displacement of fracture fragments and the associated cord compromise. CT is particularly beneficial in observing the lateral mass and posterior elements that are often more difficult to read on plain radiographs due to overlap of normal structures and the patient positioning required to obtain these views. Visualization of horizontal fractures is a serious limitation of CT. CT is limited as a modality for follow-up of soft tissue injuries inferred from X-ray as well. If MRI is not available, postmyelogram CT with a contrast agent is superior to normal CT for spinal canal analysis. Follow-up evaluation of fractures found on X-ray is enhanced with both the CT and MRI with the addition of a contrast agent.[44-46]

ISSUE REGARDING PROTECTIVE ATHLETIC EQUIPMENT

Regardless of the athlete's condition, the protective equipment will eventually need to be removed. It should be emphasized that the athlete's protective equipment should be left in place as long as possible. It is generally agreed upon that the ER, with all the emergency equipment on hand, is preferred to the playing field when removing protective equipment from the potentially spine-injured athlete.[24,47,48] It is essential that prior planning and sports emergency care team development include educating ER staff regarding sports equipment and proper equipment removal protocol to ensure that the ER is, in fact, the safest place for removal of the athlete's protective equipment. Still, the type of protective equipment used and its specific characteristics may require on-field removal. Therefore, the efficient sports emergency care team is prepared with the proper psychomotor skills and equipment required to properly prepare an athlete for transport, including facemask removal, preparation of the shoulder pads for proper transport, and complete equipment removal in the ER or on the field.

Research to date has centered on football equipment and the injured cervical spine, neglecting the unique challenges presented by other sports' protective equipment. Hockey and lacrosse equipment, for example, is not associated with the same individual fitting guidelines associated with football.[42,49-51] Therefore, this often ill-fitting equipment may not afford the sports emergency care team the same luxuries relative to aided in-line immobilization during assessment and transfer procedures. When dealing with any type of protective equipment, the sports emergency care team must assess the benefits of the presented equipment. If the protective equipment is aiding in in-line stabilization and immobilization, the equipment should be left in place as long as possible. However, if the equipment is a liability during immobilization efforts, it must be removed. An ill-fitting helmet that is left in place may hamper immobilization efforts by allowing the athlete's head to move within the helmet during log-rolling or after the athlete has been immobilized on a rigid support. Ill-fitting helmets and shoulder pads only result in immobilization of the equipment, allowing dangerous movement of the athlete's body within the equipment.

Controversy surrounding removal of athletic equipment during emergency situations has centered on the criteria for removal rather than the removal technique.[39,52] With prior facemask removal and proper preparation for transport, there are few indications for complete removal of well-fitted equipment that aids in immobilization of the athlete without hindering acute management principles. However, unique situations such as transferring an injured athlete following application of an AED may require complete equipment removal because the equipment no longer provides aid in maintaining immobilization of the athlete during transfer to a rigid support. Indications for complete equipment removal are protocol decisions that must be made by individual sports emergency care teams. However, the guiding rule regarding removal of any piece of equipment should be whether or not the piece of equipment in question is aiding in maintaining the team's primary objectives of maintaining the athlete's vital signs and maintaining in-line stabilization during transfer of the athlete to a rigid support. As long as the equipment does not hinder management of the sports emergency care team's primary objectives, it is best left in place in order to avoid unnecessary delays in transport and to minimize extraneous movement of the athlete.

It must be emphasized once again that an athlete's helmet and shoulder pads should be left in place and only removed when emergently required or following initial radiographic assessment in the ER. The sports emergency care team can all but eliminate any need to remove a protective helmet and shoulder pads from a potentially spine-injured athlete with proper planning. This level of competency must be a primary objective of every sports emergency care team member. However, as is the case with any team approach or planning process, there are always unforeseen circumstances that are impossible to predict or plan for. Some of these might indicate complete equipment removal. Therefore, it is important that the process of complete equipment removal be reviewed and practiced. These same skills are required of ER personnel who must use the same CSI precaution protocols to remove protective athletic equipment following initial radiographic assessment prior to more thorough assessment.

The following protocol is suggested when the decision to remove equipment has been made:

- If protective helmet removal is necessary:
  ❖ Team member A, maintaining immobilization of the head and neck, transfers stabilization of the head and neck to team member B. This is accomplished by having team member B position his or her hands around the athlete's neck such that his or her fingers cradle and support the cervical spine from C7 to the occiput.
  ❖ Team member A then prepares the helmet for removal by cutting the chinstraps and removing the cheek pads.
  ❖ Team member A then gently separates the helmet at the ear holes and pulls it over the top of the athlete's head while tilting the helmet forward to clear the occiput.
  ❖ Team member A then uses toweling to pack and fill the 1-inch to 2-inch gap left between the athlete's head and the ground to prevent hyperextension of the neck.
  ❖ Team member A then retakes control of the head and neck from Team member B.

If it is possible to extract the facemask prior to removing the helmet, it becomes easier to tilt the helmet anteriorly without fear of catching the facemask on the athlete's face.

- If shoulder pad removal or both helmet and shoulder pad removal is required:

  ❖ Team member A is positioned above the head of the athlete and is responsible for maintaining stabilization at all times.

  ❖ Team member B cuts through the jersey and chest straps, as well as the jersey sides and any clothing worn under the pads. Next, he or she cuts the laces on the front of the pads. When completed at the onset, these steps decrease the amount of time the head must be stabilized off the ground following helmet removal and prior to shoulder pad removal. It also reduces the number of times transfer of stabilization is required.

  ❖ Team member B then cuts the chinstrap of the helmet and pops out the cheek pads.

  ❖ Stabilization is then transferred to team member B.

  ❖ Team member A gently separates the helmet at the ear holes and pulls it over the top of the athlete's head while tilting the helmet forward to clear the occiput.

  ❖ After removing the helmet, team member A gently pulls the pads from under the athlete and applies a cervical collar.

  ❖ Team member A then resumes stabilization of the head and neck.

References

1. Otis JC, Burnstein AH, Torg SJ. Mechanisms and pathomechanics of athletic injuries to the cervical spine. In: Torg JS, ed. *Athletic Injuries to the Head, Neck, and Face*. 2nd ed. St. Louis, Mo: Mosby; 1991:438-456.

2. Boden BP, Tacchetti RL, Cantu RC, Knowles SB, Mueller FO. Catastrophic cervical spine injuries in high school and college football players. *Am J Sports Med*. 2006;34:1223-1232.

3. Tackle leaves Idaho State defensive back paralyzed. *Associated Press*. September 24, 2996:2C.

4. Bell J. Doctors: Brown got fast, effective care. *USA Today*. December 23, 1997:1C.

5. Torg J. Prevention of cervical spine injuries. Presentation at: Adam Taliaferro Foundation Medical Workshop; September 19, 2006; Voorhees, NJ.

6. Heck JF, Clarke KS, Peterson TR, Torg JS, Weis MP. National Athletic Trainers' Association Position Statement: head-down contact and spearing in tackle football. *Journal of Athletic Training*. 2004;39:101-111.

7. Otis JC. Biomechanics of spine injury. In: Cantu RC, ed. *Neurologic Athletic Head and Spine Injuries*. Philadelphia: WB Saunders; 2000:6-21.

8. Swartz EE, Floyd RT, Cendoma MJ. Cervical spine functional anatomy and the biomechanics of injury due to compressive loading. *Journal of Athletic Training.* 2006;40:155-161.

9. Heck J. The incidence of spearing during a high school's 1975 and 1990 football seasons. *Journal of Athletic Training.* 1996;31(1):31-36.

10. Cantu RC, Meuller FO. Catastrophic spine injuries in football (1977-1989). *J Spinal Disord.* 1990;3:227-231.

11. Cantu RC, Meuller FO. Catastrophic football injuries: 1977-1998. *Neurosurgery.* 2000;47:673-675, discussion 675-677.

12. Buchanan LE, Nawoczenski D. An overview. In: Buchanan LE, Nawoczenski D, eds. *Spinal Cord Injury: Concepts and Management Approaches.* Baltimore, Md: Williams & Wilkins; 1987:11-18.

13. Riser TV, Mudiyam R, Waters RL. Orthopedic evaluation of spinal cord injury and management of vertebral fractures. In: Adkins HV, ed. *Spinal Cord Injury.* New York: Churchill Livingstone; 1985:1-36.

14. Wilberger JE. Athletic cervical spinal cord and spine injuries. In: Cantu RC, ed. *Neurologic Athletic Head and Spine Injuries.* Philadelphia: WB Saunders Company; 2000:144-152.

15. Podolsky S, Baraff LJ, Simon RR, Hoffman JR, Larmon B, Ablon W. Efficacy of cervical spine immobilization methods. *J Trauma.* 1983;23:461-465.

16. Waters RL, Apple DF, Meyer PR, Cotler JM, Adkins RH. Emergency and acute management of spinal trauma. In: Stover SL, DeLisa JA, Whiteneck GG, eds. *Spinal Cord Injury: Clinical Outcomes From the Model Systems.* Gaithersburg, Md: Aspen; 1995:21-25.

17. Go BK, DeVivo MJ, Richards SJ. The epidemiology of spinal cord injury. In: Stover SL, DeLisa JA, Whiteneck GG, eds. *Spinal Cord Injury: Clinical Outcomes From the Model Systems.* Gaithersburg, Md: Aspen; 1995:26-55.

18. Polumbo MA, Hulstyn MJ, Fadale PD, O'Brien T, Shall L. The effect of protective football equipment on alignment of the injured cervical spine. *Am J Sports Med.* 1996;24(4):446-452.

19. Vegso JJ, Torg JS. Field evaluation and management of cervical spine injuries. In: Torg JS, ed. *Athletic Injuries to the Head, Neck, and Face.* 2nd ed. St. Louis, Mo: Mosby; 1991:426-437.

20. Schubert A. Spinal cord trauma. Available from: http://www.anes.ccf.org:8080/ PILOT/NEURO/sci.htm. Accessed September 9, 1997.

21. American Red Cross. Injuries. In: *Standard First Aid.* St. Louis, Mo: Mosby; 1993.

22. Feld F. Management of the critically injured football player. *Journal of Athletic Training.* 1993;28(3):206-212.

23. Ray R, Lunchies C, Bazuin D, Farrell R. Airway preparation techniques for the cervical spine-injured football player. *Journal of Athletic Training.* 1995;30(3):217-221.

24. Kleiner DM, Almquist JL, Bailes J, et al. *Prehospital Care of the Spine-Injured Athlete. A document From the Inter-Association Task Force for Appropriate Care of the Spine-Injured Athlete.* Dallas, TX: Inter-Association Task Force for the Appropriate Care of the Spine-Injured Athlete; 2001.

25. Block JJ, Kleiner DM, Knox KE. Football helmet facemask removal with various tools and straps. *Journal of Athletic Training.* 1995;31(Suppl. 2, Abstract No. 7):11.

26. Kleiner DM. Facemask removal vs facemask retraction. *Journal of Athletic Training.* 1995;31(Suppl. 2):32.

27. Knox KE, Kleiner DM. EMT shears effectiveness for facemask removal. *Journal of Athletic Training.* 1995;31(Suppl. 2):17.

28. Rehberg SR. Rating facemask removal tools. *NATA News.* January 1995:26-27.

29. Swartz EE, Armstrong CW, Rankin JM, Rodgers B. A 3-dimensional analysis of facemask removal tools in inducing helmet movement. *Journal of Athletic Training.* 2002;37:178-184.

30. Decoster LC, Shirley CP, Swartz EE. Football face-mask removal with a cordless screwdriver on helmets used for at least one season of play. *Journal of Athletic Training.* 2005;40:169-173.

31. Gosch HH, Gooding E, Schneider RC. An experimental study of cervical spine and cord injuries. *J Trauma.* 1972;12:570.

32. Hanak M, Scott A. *Spinal Cord Injury: An Illustrated Guide for Health Care Professionals.* New York: Springer; 1983:24-33.

33. Waninger KN. Management of the helmeted athlete with suspected CSI. *Am J Sports Med.* 2004;32:1331-1350.

34. Swartz EE, Norkus SA, Cappaert T, Decoster LC. Football equipment design affects facemask removal efficiency. *Am J Sports Med.* 2005;33:1210-1219.

35. Donaldson WF, Lauerman WC, Heil B, Blanc R, Swenson T. Helmet and shoulder pad removal from a player with a suspected cervical spine injury: a cadaveric model. *Spine.* 1998;23(16):1729-1732.

36. Banerjee R, Palumbo MA, Fadale PD. Catastrophic cervical spine injuries in the collision sport athlete: part 2: principles of emergency care. *Am J Sports Med.* 2004;32:1760-1764.

37. Delbridge TR, Auble TE, Garrison HG, Menegazzi JJ. Discomfort in healthy volunteer immobilized on wooden backboards and vacuum mattress splints. *Prehospital Disaster Med.* 1993;8(2):S63.

38. Del Rossi G, Horodyski M, Powers ME. A comparison of spine board transfer techniques and the effect of training on performance. *Journal of Athletic Training.* 2003;38:204-208.

39. Segan RD, Cassidy C, Bentkowski J. A discussion of the issue of football helmet removal and suspected cervical spine injuries. *Journal of Athletic Training.* 1993;28(4):294-305.

40. Lovell ME, Evans JH. A comparison of spinal board and the vacuum stretcher, spinal stability and interface pressure. *Injury.* 1994;25(3):7-8.

41. Johnson DR, Hauswald M, Stockhoff CY. Comparison of a vacuum splint device to a rigid backboard for spinal immobilization. *Am J Emerg Med.* 1996;14(4):369-372.

42. Prinsen RK, Syrotuik DG, Reid DC. Position of the cervical vertebrae during helmet removal and cervical collar application in football and hockey. *Clin J Sport Med.* 1995;5(3):155-161.

43. Cendoma MJ. Evaluation of various facemask removal techniques. *NATA News.* April 2006:14-18.

44. Jahre C, Pavlov H, Deck MDF. Commuted tomography and magnetic imaging of cervical spine trauma. In: Torg JS, ed. *Athletic Injuries to the Head, Neck, and Face.* 2nd ed. St. Louis, Mo: Mosby; 1991:412-425.

45. Pavlov H. Radiographic evaluation of the cervical spine and related structures. In: Torg JS, ed. *Athletic Injuries to the Head, Neck, and Face.* 2nd ed. St. Louis, Mo: Mosby; 1991:384-411.

46. Wales LP, Knopp RK, Morishima MS. Recommendations for evaluation of the acutely injured cervical spine: a radiologic algorithm. *Ann Emerg Med.* 1980;9:422-428.

47. Swenson TM, Lauerman WC, Blanc RO, Donaldson WF. Cervical spine alignment in the immobilized football player. Radiographic analysis before and after helmet removal. *Am J Sports Med.* 1997;25(2):226-230.

48. Waninger KN. On-field management of potential cervical spine injury in helmeted football players: leave the helmet on! *Clin J Sport Med.* 1998;8(2):124-129.

49. Metz CM, Kuhn JE, Greenfield ML. Cervical spine alignment in immobilized hockey players: radiographic analysis with and without helmets and shoulder pads. *Clin J Sport Med.* 1998;8(2):92-95.

50. Sherbondy PS, Hertel JN, Sebastianelli WJ. The effect of protective equipment on cervical spine alignment in collegiate lacrosse players. *Am J Sports Med.* 2006;34:1675-1679.

51. LaPrade RF, Schnetzler KA, Broxerman RJ, Wentorf F, Wendland E, Gilbert TJ. Cervical spine alignment in the immobilized ice hockey player: a computed tomographic analysis of the effects of helmet removal. *Am J Sports Med.* 2000;28:800-803.

52. Bronus S. Put me in the game, coach. *J Emerg Med Srvc.* 1993;18(2):26-37.

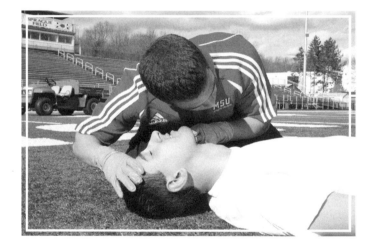

Chapter 7 — *Unconsciousness and Seizures*

David A. Middlemas, EdD, ATC

"Are you all right? Can you hear me?" These are 2 questions for which sports emergency care personnel always hope the answer is "yes." Changes in a person's level of consciousness (LOC) can range from mild disorientation or confusion to unconsciousness. Changes in LOC indicate impairment of normal brain function or brain injury in almost every instance. Emergencies in the athletic venue resulting in changes in the victim's state of consciousness can occur from injury events or changes in brain function as a result of a medical condition or disease.

This chapter will focus on the causes of unconsciousness and seizure events. We will also learn the strategies and methods of recognizing and caring for victims of emergencies involving changes in LOC and/or seizures.

The Athlete Is Down and Does Not Respond!

When an athlete is down on the field or court and does not respond, sports emergency care personnel must determine the potential reasons the victim is unconscious and take actions to stabilize the victim and prevent further injury. Loss of consciousness can happen as a result of an injury or a crisis resulting from a medical condition. It is important to know the events that caused the athlete to become unconscious because they are essential in determining the course of care for this individual.

The unconscious victim presents a challenge during the process of patient assessment because he or she is not able to provide the sports team professional with the verbal feedback normally used to determine the extent of injury or illness. In the best of situations, sports emergency care personnel are in a position to observe the events preceding the athlete's becoming unconscious. They would be able to see any contact or collision that caused the injury or to witness the victim's collapse. Witnessing what happened provides the caregiver with information that directs the course of care.

Unfortunately, in the world of youth, scholastic, and collegiate athletics, sports emergency care personnel cannot be present at all events. There are many venues in which multiple practices or contests are held concurrently in different locations. Help may be summoned and arrive at the scene of the emergency after the fact. In this situation, information about the events leading up to the incident must be collected without the victim's input or the luxury of witnessing the collapse. Sports emergency care personnel must observe the environment in which the athlete became unconscious and the position in which he or she is found to begin piecing together what happened and the possible extent of injury or illness.

As in any other emergency, conducting a primary survey to determine the presence of life-threatening conditions and the stability of the victim is the first order of business. It is a good premise to adopt the mindset to assume the worst and hope for the best. Athletes who become unconscious during practice or competition are often involved in some sort of contact or collision. Immediate immobilization of the spine and head is always warranted in unobserved athletic emergencies resulting in unconsciousness, even when the cause may not appear to be a result of contact. In so doing, you will always protect the victim from things that could make the condition worse while completing your assessment. Aggravation of a possible spinal fracture could result in temporary or permanent paralysis, deterioration of vital signs, loss of consciousness, or death.

Initial patient assessment should follow the ABC Sx3 format discussed in Chapter 3. If the athlete is responsive, he or she has an airway, is breathing, and has blood circulating through the body, evaluate the Airway status, assess the presence and quality of the victim's Breathing, and check for Circulation. If the athlete is not responsive, the athletic trainer must be prepared to provide basic life support in the event breathing and/or pulse have stopped.

The assessment of breathing and pulse should usually be done in the position in which the athlete is found. Athletes will often be found lying on their side or face down after a collision or incident that would cause unconsciousness during practice or a game. Evaluating the athlete in the position in which he or she is found will allow you to determine the presence of breathing and pulse without potentially aggravating possible head or neck injuries. In addition, if the athlete is unconscious, leaving him or her prone or sidelying will provide the same protection to a patent airway as having the victim in the recovery position. Initial assessment of responsiveness, breathing, and pulse in victims of possible unconsciousness that is not a result of collision or trauma should also be performed in the position in which the victim is found.

When the athlete does not respond or the response is so incoherent or diminished that it is obvious that he or she is in distress, EMS should be activated immediately. Because the amount of time it takes for EMS to arrive varies, athletic trainers must be prepared to continue to monitor vital signs and provide basic life support in the event breathing and/or pulse stop. Pulse rate and quality, respiration rate and quality, blood pressure, and other vital signs should be assessed and the results recorded at 5-min intervals while waiting for EMS to arrive.

Evaluation of the patient's level of consciousness should also be included in the assessment. One of the common tools to evaluate the quality of a person's responses is the Glasgow Coma Scale.[1] This easy to administer scale evaluates an individual's response to stimuli, the quality of verbal responses, and ability to move. Its use is presented later in this chapter.

The information from the patient assessment should be given to the paramedic or EMT as part of the process of patient transfer. When a collision or other contact is part of the mechanism of injury or there is other reason to suspect possible cervical injury, the athlete's head and spine should be immobilized while waiting for the ambulance. The methods and procedures for these situations are covered in Chapter 6.

Understanding Loss of Consciousness

Changes in the level of consciousness can range from completely aware, responsive, and functional to unconscious, unresponsive, and pretty much anywhere in between. In this section, we will explain some of the common causes of unconsciousness that may be seen in the sports medicine environment. Some of these are related to injury and some are not. Having a better understanding of the common causes of unconsciousness and types of conditions you may encounter will help you to decide what actions to take.

SYNCOPE

Sometimes an individual may pass out without any immediately obvious reason. Syncope occurs when someone becomes unconscious and recovers quickly without assistance. Common names for syncope include "fainting," "passing out," "collapsing," or a "blackout." These episodes are usually accompanied by loss of voluntary muscle tone, hence the victim stumbles or falls to the floor if standing or slumps forward in a chair if sitting.

Victims of syncope may have changes in vital signs similar to someone in shock. In addition to becoming unresponsive, the patient may present with pale skin that may be cool to the touch, rapid weak pulse, increase in breathing rate, and drop in blood pressure. For example, an individual having a syncopal episode may have pale skin, a weak pulse at the rate of 110 beats per minute, irregular breathing at the rate of 24 breaths per minute, and a blood pressure of 90/60 mm Hg. All of these symptoms are consistent with conditions in which blood flow to the brain is diminished.

By its very definition, when someone has a syncopal episode (passes out), the condition is often temporary and the victim usually recovers on his or her own without medical assistance. It is possible that he or she may only have a partial loss of consciousness, becoming disoriented, confused, and lightheaded and temporarily lose awareness of his or her surroundings. More benign causes of syncopal episodes include upsetting emotional events, psychogenic shock, response to illness (ie, cold or flu), or orthostatic hypotension. Syncope can also be caused by more serious conditions that cause diminished blood flow to the brain, including dehydration and cardiogenic shock.

Syncope is a common cause for emergency room visits. Syncope should be considered as a potential diagnosis in any situation where there is an unexplained fall or unexplained brief loss of consciousness, especially if the individual becomes alert and aware shortly after the incident. The return of awareness after collapse is also consistent with the return of blood flow to the brain when the patient becomes horizontal. Recovery is usually spontaneous in many cases. Emergency care for the condition involves protecting the victim from injury during the collapse and assessment for significant injury or illness. It is common for individuals to refuse EMS or medical treatment after recovering from a syncopal episode. Reasons for refusing medical care may include embarrassment, the person feeling as though he or she has returned to normal, or the possibility that this has happened before in response to emotionally traumatic events. Regardless, sports emergency care personnel should be thorough in their assessment, taking the time to rule out any serious underlying cause for the episode.

STUPOR

Stupor is defined as a decreased state of mental activity or awareness that can be associated with drowsiness or diminished response. One possible description of stupor is that it is short of unconsciousness and the patient can be awakened or will respond to the stimuli. It is possible that someone who is stuporous will respond to the rescuer but will then return to his or her state of disorientation or semiconsciousness. The response may be incoherent or appear disoriented. As always, the need for emergency care directly relates to the stability of the patient's vital signs, the amount of disorientation, and the difficulty in arousing the patient. When an individual is difficult to arouse, provides incoherent responses, and/or returns to the semiconscious state after being aroused, EMS should be activated for care and transportation to an emergency room.

Stupor can occur as a result of head injury or secondary to shock. It can also be a symptom of drug or alcohol abuse, advanced heat illness, insulin shock, or hyperglycemia. It is important to determine the underlying cause of stupor in active individuals who become semiconscious or drowsy, which may also require emergency care and/or psychological intervention.

COMA

Coma is defined as a deep state of unconsciousness during which the patient does not react or respond to stimuli in the environment. Individuals who are comatose do not respond to verbal, visual, tactile, or painful stimuli. It is not unusual for someone in a coma to have a Glasgow score of E = 1, V = 1, M = 3, or a total of 5 or less. Someone who becomes comatose has suffered serious loss of brain function. Coma can often happen as a result of serious head injury or after consuming large amounts of alcohol or drugs. Coma can also occur after severe diabetic reaction or hemorrhage in the brain. Although not seen frequently in the athletic venue, the possibility of an athlete suffering deep unconsciousness after a head injury is real. In sports such as soccer, ice hockey, and rugby, in which high-force collisions occur between athletes' heads or in high-speed events such as equestrian, motocross, or racing, athletes have the real possibility of significant head injury from collisions or falls. "Extreme sports" such as freestyle skateboarding and snowboarding, BMX events, half pipe skate, bike, and snow sports have gained popularity with recreational and club participants in recent years. These activities all involve aerial stunts from which participants, even when wearing a helmet, can suffer head trauma resulting in unconsciousness. Athletic trainers and other medical personnel must be prepared to provide basic life support in the event of unconsciousness due to injury.

HEAD TRAUMA

In many athletic activities, the participants are exposed to contact and collisions leading to the possibility of head injury during the normal course of play. Sports like football, ice hockey, motor sports, lacrosse, baseball, and softball require that players wear protective helmets while participating. On the other hand, helmets are not required in many other activities in which collisions and falls occur regularly, including soccer, rugby, wrestling, gymnastics, rodeo, and recreational skiing and snowboarding. Incidents involving head injuries and unconsciousness have occurred in all of these sports.

When a victim is unconscious immediately after a fall or collision, the sports medicine team member must assume that there is significant head injury and the high possibility of spinal injury. Immediate on-the-field spinal immobilization, assessment of vital signs, and preparation for the possibility of providing basic life support are paramount. EMS must be called immediately and the athlete should be only removed from the playing area on a spineboard by ambulance.

Unconsciousness does not always happen immediately when an athlete suffers a head injury. There are times when the injury in the brain that results from a head injury is the result of bleeding within the skull. If the bleeding continues long enough to place enough pressure on the brain tissue within the skull, the victim's neurological status will begin to worsen. It is often the speed at which the neurological signs and symptoms change that provides the best indicator of the severity of the bleeding. Details on intracranial injuries are presented in Chapter 8.

Assessment of the Athlete With Loss of Consciousness

Assessment of the athlete's responsiveness involves more than just seeing whether or not he or she responds to you; it also involves determining the quality and coherence of that response. The role of the sports emergency care personnel in this situation is to assess the athlete for diminished or abnormal brain function by evaluating basic neurological functions such as dizziness, balance, vision, eye movement, memory, and the ability to speak.

Abnormal brain function can occur as a result of a number of conditions, such as trauma, a decrease in oxygenated blood supply to the brain, or a neurological disorder. Hence, assessing brain function is essential when assessing an athlete who has suddenly become unconscious. Although abnormal brain function is most commonly associated with trauma, this chapter will focus on atraumatic causes. Detailed information on the recognition and management of traumatic brain injury is covered in Chapter 8.

A tool commonly used to assess neurological status in serious injury or illness is the Glasgow Coma Scale.[1] The scale is broken into 3 components— eye-opening response (E), verbal response (V), and motor response (M). The victim is scored in each of the 3 categories, adding the 3 scores to give a total score. Because these 3 types of activities are important indicators of quality of brain function and neurological status, the scores in each of the individual categories and the total Glasgow Coma Score are reported. The administration of the Glasgow Coma Scale and its scoring are summarized in Table 7-1. The scale can be a useful tool in assessing the severity of the condition of an athlete who is unconscious or who is experiencing an altered level of consciousness. Glasgow scores are reported in the format E + V + M = Total Score. Simply reporting the total does not provide the physician with information as to which categories had stronger or weaker performance by the patient. Reporting the score on each section and the total gives insight as to the nature of neurological deficit for the individual patient. Generally speaking, a total Glasgow score between 13 and 15 would indicate mild brain injury, 9 to 12 would indicate moderate brain injury, and a total of 8 or less would indicate significant loss of normal brain function.

Table 7-1

GLASGOW COMA SCALE

Total = E + V + M

Eye Opening (4)	Verbal (5)	Motor Response (6)
4 = Spontaneous	5 = Normal conversation	6 = Normal
3 = To voice	4 = Disoriented conversation	5 = Localizes to pain
2 = To pain	3 = Words, incoherent	4 = Withdraws to pain
1 = None	2 = No words, only sounds	3 = Decorticate posture
	1 = None	2 = Decerebrate
		1 = None

Amnesia is the inability to accurately remember information. It is important to determine whether amnesia is present in individuals with head injury or significantly altered brain function by asking the victim questions to which he or she should know the answers. It is also important to remember to ask questions to which the interviewer knows the answer; otherwise it may be impossible to determine whether the athlete is answering appropriately. For example, asking the athlete questions about what he or she ate for breakfast may not be a question to which the interviewer will know the answer. Questions referring to place ("Do you know where you are?"), time ("What is the date?" "Approximately what time is it?"), person ("Can you tell me your name? Do you remember my name?"), and event ("What are you doing here? What team are you playing?") are all appropriate questions to which the interviewer and the athlete should know the answer.

There are 2 types of amnesia for which you should assess the athlete on the field. Retrograde amnesia is the inability to remember events before the time of the injury. Anterograde amnesia (sometimes referred to as post-traumatic amnesia) is the inability to remember events after the time of injury. When dealing with victims suffering memory loss, it is important to continue to reassess memory function at frequent intervals. This is done to see if there are any changes that could indicate the injury or condition is worsening with time. Worsening anterograde amnesia could be an indication of intracranial bleeding, which is an emergency. Table 7-2 gives examples of the types of questions one might ask to assess memory loss.

It is also important to perform a physical examination that is focused on evaluating the status of brain function. In addition to the things discussed above, assessing the victim for headache, vision, pupillary response, eye

Table 7-2

ASSESSMENT OF MEMORY LOSS

Retrograde Amnesia	Anterograde Amnesia
Ask questions about information or events occurring before the injury	Ask questions about information or events after the injury
What is your name? What were you doing before you got hit? Where are you? What day is it? Who am I?	Provide a list of unrelated words to remember: Light Spoon Flower Radio Dog

movement, facial muscles, tongue motion, and ability to speak clearly provide feedback on brain function. Because these activities are controlled directly by the brain through cranial nerves, any abnormalities are very likely indications of injury or damage to the brain. Refer to Chapter 8 for additional information on assessing cranial nerve function.

Serious or critical injuries or medical emergencies affecting the brain can result in significant damage to the portions of the brain controlling motor function. Although these situations rarely occur in the athletic venue, it is very important that the sports medicine team member recognize the signs of these emergencies. When serious brain damage occurs, the victim may present in one of two abnormal positions or postures indicating significant damage to the brain. Decorticate posturing is identified by flexion of the fingers, wrists, and elbows with the forearms on the chest. The legs are extended and rotated slightly inward. Decorticate posturing indicates damage along the pathway controlling messages from the cortex of the brain to the spinal cord. Patient position occurs because the mechanisms that inhibit flexion of the upper extremities and extension of the lower extremities have been damaged. Decerebrate posturing presents with both the upper and lower extremities in extended positions. The arms will be at the patient's sides and the neck will be arched into extension. Decerebrate posture in the unconscious patient indicates possible damage to the brainstem, which is more serious than that indicated by the decorticate posture. It is possible for a patient to go from decorticate to decerebrate over time as the patient's brain condition worsens. Both positions are presented in Figure 7-1.

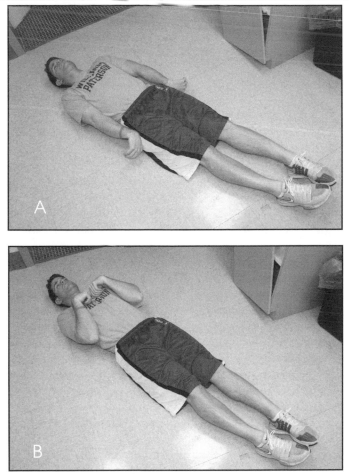

Figure 7-1. (A) Decerebrate posturing. (B) Decorticate posturing.

There will be times when an athlete may present with minor or minimal changes in the signs and symptoms related to brain function. The changes could be a result of an injury or a medically related problem. Unfortunately, the world of sports is not immune to problems resulting from substance abuse or medical crises that lead to unconsciousness. Key factors in determining the urgency of the situation include the neurological status of the patient, whether it is stable or changing, and the length of time the symptoms have been present. In situations in which the changes are relatively minor and stable, the athlete can see his or her physician for evaluation. If there is doubt as to the individual's safety or medical stability, EMS should be activated. In either event, the athlete should not be allowed to return to activity until cleared by a physician.

Seizures

Changes in a person's LOC may be due to the occurrence of sudden, uncontrolled, abnormal electrical activity in the brain. This condition may present itself in different ways. Depending on where in the brain the abnormal activity takes place, the victim can have a blank stare, minor twitches, convulsions, and/or unconsciousness. Seizures can be caused by a number of problems, including epilepsy, head injury, fever, poisoning, and insulin shock (hypoglycemia). The causes of seizures may not be determined in as many as 50% of the individuals having one.

The athlete is said to have a generalized seizure when abnormal electrical activity takes place throughout the entire brain. Because the entire brain is involved, the patient is likely to become unresponsive and unaware of surroundings, become unconscious, and collapse. The most common type of generalized seizure is the tonic-clonic, or grand mal seizure. The tonic phase involves stiffening of the muscles of the body, at which point the victim will collapse. There will be muscle spasms and convulsions of the limbs after the tonic phase; this is called the clonic phase. The seizure will end after a couple of minutes. The person will be tired, potentially irritable for a short time, and is said to be postictal.

Efforts should not be made to restrain someone having convulsions because it is not possible to stop the seizure and injury to the victim or rescuer can occur. The primary focus in providing emergency care for an athlete having a seizure is to protect him or her from injury and to monitor vital signs and condition until he or she has regained consciousness and awareness (Figure 7-2). Although it may appear that the victim is not breathing during a seizure, there is sufficient air exchange. After the seizure ends, the athletic trainer should be in a position to provide support and assistance as the patient reorients to the environment and deals with any embarrassment.

A partial seizure happens when only part of the brain is affected by the abnormal electrical activity. In this case, spasm will be limited to the area controlled by the affected part of the brain. In the case of a partial seizure, the victim will most likely not lose consciousness and should recover fairly quickly on his or her own.

When the athlete has a partial seizure that generalizes into a grand mal seizure, it will usually be preceded by an aura, which is a period of altered sensation before the onset of the seizure. The individual may describe flashing lights; a feeling of warmth; or unusual sights, smells, or tastes before the seizure begins. The aura serves as a warning to individuals with a seizure disorder that a seizure is imminent, providing time to sit down or get to a location to minimize injury from the seizure.

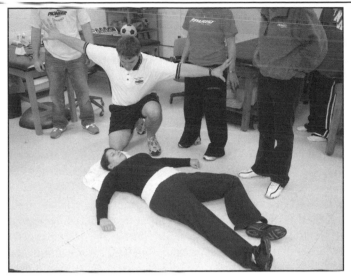

Figure 7-2. Protecting the seizure patient.

When an individual has a seizure disorder such as epilepsy, he or she is usually aware of the signs of oncoming seizure and the sequence of events that take place during a seizure. In such cases, management of the situation during the seizure is the primary concern of the caregiver, and EMS may not be indicated. For such individuals, the primary causes of seizure are usually forgetting to take seizure medication, physical or emotional stress, or underlying illness. The athlete will recover spontaneously without significant incident in a matter of a few minutes in the vast majority of situations.

Seizures are an emergency situation when they last longer than 5 min, when they repeat without the person regaining consciousness in between, if the victim is injured during the seizure, or if the person does not return to normal consciousness and alertness afterward. The condition in which a seizure continues or repeats over a period of at least 30 min is sometimes called status epilepticus. It indicates ongoing abnormal seizure activity in the brain and requires emergency medical intervention.

When a seizure takes place after head injury or as a result of a medical emergency, EMS should be activated immediately and the sports emergency care provider must be prepared to provide support for breathing and pulse. Brain damage from head trauma, poisoning, insulin shock, or other medical emergency can be significant and life threatening. Any information the sports emergency care provider can provide to the physician will be important in determining the nature and extent of brain injury and the course of care.

Other Points to Consider

Concerns sometimes arise regarding the participation of individuals with conditions such as epilepsy or other seizure disorders in sports. Anyone with an underlying medical condition that can result in altered states of consciousness or brain function should consult his or her physician before attempting new, demanding activities. In general, individuals whose epilepsy or seizure disorder is not controlled should refrain from sports or activities that could increase the chances of a seizure occurring. A seizure disorder is considered under control when the athlete is taking the appropriate medication as ordered by a physician and has been seizure-free for a period of time determined by the doctor.

Certain activities that could significantly increase the possibility of a seizure, such as boxing, should be avoided. Activities in which serious injury could result if an individual had a seizure during the activity, such as rock climbing or sky diving, may also be contraindicated for some individuals. On the other hand, many contact sports, like lacrosse, hockey, and possibly football, may be allowed with physician consent. In these cases, it is essential that the athlete has the proper protective equipment and that it fits properly. The sports medicine team must work together to ensure a safe playing situation for the athlete concerned. Epilepsy and other neurological disorders are not necessarily grounds for disqualification from sports or physical activity.

References

1. Teasdale G, Jennett B. Assessment of coma and impaired consciousness: a practical scale. *Lancet.* 1974,2:81-84.

Bibliography

American Red Cross. *Emergency Response 1995 USDOT First Responder Curriculum.* Yardley, Pa: Staywell Publishing; 2001.

Booher JM, Thibodeau GA. *Athletic Injury Assessment.* 4th ed. New York: McGraw Hill; 2000.

Ebell MH. Syncope: initial evaluation and prognosis (Point-of-Care Guides). *Am Fam Physician.* 2006;74(8):1367.

Guskiewicz KM, Bruce SL, Cantu RC, et al. National Athletic Trainers' Association position abatement: management of sport-related concussion. *Journal of Athletic Training.* 2004;39(3):280-297.

Harmon KG. Assessment and Management of Concussion in Sports. *American Family Physician.* Available at: http://www.afp.org/afp/990901ap/887.html. Accessed September 22, 2006.

Luke A, Micheli L. Sports injuries: emergency assessment and field-side care. *Pediatr Rev.* 1999;20:291-300.

Moyer C. Using the Glasgow Coma Scale: for accurate results, experience counts. *Am J Nurs.* 1991;91(7):14

National Registry of Emergency Medical Technicians. Advanced Level Practical Examination; PATIENT ASSESSMENT – TRAUMA. National Registry of Emergency Medical Technicians, Inc, Columbus, Ohio. 2000. Available at: http://www.nremt.org/downloads/Patient%20Trauma.pdf Accessed October 14, 2006.

Pollak AN, ed. *Emergency Care and Transportation of the Sick and Injured.* 9th ed. Boston, Mass: Jones and Bartlett Publishers; 2005.

Prentice WE. *Arnheim's Principles of Athletic Training.* 12th ed. New York: McGraw Hill; 2006.

Spitz MC, Towbin B, Honigman B, Shantz D. Emergency seizure care in adults with known epilepsy. *Journal of Epilepsy.* 1996;9(3):15-465.

Valente LR. Seizures and epilepsy. *Clinician Reviews.* 2000;10(3):79.

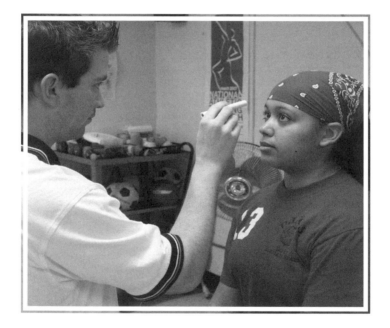

Management of Traumatic Brain Injury

Chapter **8**

Michael J. Cendoma, MS, ATC and Robb S. Rehberg, PhD, ATC, CSCS, NREMT

The burden of responsibility for providing a safe environment for sports participation falls, in part, on the sports emergency care personnel charged with the care, prevention, and management of sports-related concussion (SRC). In past years, management of SRCs has been, perhaps, the most frustrating and confusing aspect of sports medicine. Research indicates that athletes in the United States suffer nearly 300,000 annual concussions. As many as 34% of the athletes suffering a concussion may not seek the care of a sports medicine professional, while 55% will receive out-patient care only.[1] It has been well established that the onset of significant signs and symptoms of SRC may not be readily observable for hours, days, or weeks following trauma.[2,3] Therefore, as many as 89% of the nearly 300,000 annual concussions suffered by athletes in the United States may not be receiving the level of care that sports medicine professionals have come to accept as minimal standards. As few as 0.021% of high school athletes will make a NCAA varsity team while only 0.00007% of athletes will make a professional team.[4] Those athletes that do make it to professional football can expect their career to last an average of 4.2 years.[5] Assuming that a football player makes a professional team and plays for an average of 4.2 years, the individual's athletic career would be finished around 26 years of age, leaving the remainder of the individual's life to be affected by complications of SRC due to improper management during his or her career. As sports emergency care personnel charged with providing the safest environment possible for athletic participation, it is unacceptable to oversee an environment that may place children and young adults at risk of a lifetime of disability resulting from such a relatively brief period of their lives as athletes.

Research in the area of SRC is providing sports emergency care personnel with valuable new knowledge that can help reduce the percentage of athletes that may be exposed to life-long complications resulting from SRC. This chapter will draw on more recent advances in knowledge pertaining to SRC to develop a practical approach for sports emergency care personnel to apply to acute management. The chapter begins with a brief overview of clinically relevant anatomy as a background that is used to develop a more sensitive acute assessment. The chapter then provides a practical approach to acute assessment of SRC.

Review of Clinically Relevant Anatomy

A review of clinically relevant anatomy is particularly relevant prior to discussions pertaining to acute care and management of SRC because a comprehensive understanding of the anatomy and function of the central nervous system (CNS) allows the sports health care professional to engage in more directed subjective assessment that is beneficial in determining the anatomical structures likely to be involved in any trauma as well as the possibility of functional deficits that may ensue.

The brain is composed of 3 major divisions: the cerebrum, the cerebellum, and the brainstem. The cerebrum is formed by the union of the right and left hemispheres of the brain. The boundary between the right and left hemisphere is defined by the longitudinal cerebral fissure located between the medial surfaces of the two hemispheres.[6,7] The hemispheres of the cerebrum are divided into 4 lobes: the frontal, parietal, occipital, and temporal. Each of the 4 lobes is defined by folds and grooves referred to as fissures or sulci.

The frontal lobe of the cerebrum spans from the foremost part of the brain to the central sulcus. The frontal lobe is responsible for motor control involving voluntary skeletal muscles as well as personality, concentration, and complex problem solving.[8] Below the frontal lobe is the lateral sulcus, marking the boundary between the superior frontal lobe and the inferior temporal lobe. The temporal lobe gathers and interprets sensory information from the ears, nose, and mouth. The occipital lobe lies near the posterior aspect of the cerebral hemisphere. Cells of the occipital lobe gather information from the optic nerve to interpret information related to vision. The occipital lobe also combines visual information with other sensory experiences. The boundary between the occipital lobe and the parietal lobe is marked on the medial aspect of the hemispheres by the parieto-occipital sulcus. The parietal lobe controls general sensory function, including temperature, pressure, pain, and proprioception. Additionally, the parietal lobe manages the understanding of speech.

The cerebellum lies immediately inferior to the posterior portions of the cerebral hemispheres and within the posterior cranial fossa.[8] The primary function of the cerebellum is unconscious coordination of muscular movement and helping to control the contraction of voluntary muscles. There are no conscious centers in the cerebellum. The cerebellum receives, evaluates, and manages information from the cerebrum, muscle spindles, and Golgi tendon organs that regulate muscle tone, equilibrium, and posture.[7] This information is then passed along to the appropriate muscle groups to regulate contractions with respect to time and strength so that a desired movement is carried out in a smooth and coordinated fashion. Injury to the cerebellum, therefore, may affect balance and voluntary movement.

The remaining sections of the brain are hidden by the cerebral hemispheres and cerebellum such that they are not readily observable. Collectively these parts of the brain are referred to as the brainstem. The brainstem constituents include the medulla oblongata, pons varolii, midbrain, and tweenbrain.[5] This region of the brain connects the cerebrum to the spinal cord and transmits messages regarding reflex control of breathing, heart rate, and blood pressure.

It should become evident that many of the questions associated with clinical assessment of SRC are actually assessments of various components of the CNS. Armed with an understanding of the location and function of various CNS structures, the sports medicine professional can determine which areas of the CNS may have been affected and as a result ask more specific questions regarding the function of the areas of the CNS that are at greatest risk of injury. The result of more specific questioning is likely a more sensitive assessment that provides the sports emergency care team with a better opportunity to uncover more subtle signs and symptoms of complications resulting from trauma to the CNS.

PROTECTION OF THE BRAIN

The following discussion regarding clinically relevant anatomy addresses anatomical structures that protect the brain from external forces. The scalp, skull, meninges, and ventricles protect the brain and CNS in various and interesting ways.

The scalp offers the first line of defense of the CNS system from external forces. External forces about the head are dissipated and absorbed by the scalp. Imagine the scalp as a loosely fit piece of 0.25-inch high-density foam atop the skull. Like a piece of foam, the scalp absorbs external forces through compression and dissipates force by moving about the cranium, aiding in prevention of injury to the brain and bones of the skull.[8]

The skull is the second line of protection for the brain. The primary functions of the bones of the cranium are to support and protect the brain, excluding the 6 ossicles of the ear.[6] The cranium includes the occipital, 2 parietal, the frontal, 2 temporal, the ethmoid, and the sphenoid bones.

The next line of defense protecting the CNS from external forces is the meninges, a continuous membrane that encases and protects both the spinal cord and the brain. The primary responsibilities of this layer are to direct forces away from the neural tissues and provide a corridor for the passage of nerves, blood vessels, and lymph vessels. The superficial most layer of the meninges is the dura. The dura mater is directly connected to the skull as it forms the internal periosteum. This vascular layer is the toughest of the meningeal layers, adding a great deal to the protective qualities of the meninges in both the cranium and the spinal column. Beyond the dura mater is the subdural space, which consists of a thin film of fluid separating the dura from the arachnoid mater. The arachnoid mater is a web-like membrane that is composed of elastic and collagenous fibers. The corresponding subarachnoid space that separates the arachnoid mater from the pia mater houses the cerebral spinal fluid (CSF), which serves to bathe and protect the brain. The pia mater is a highly vascularized membrane that closely adheres to the fissures and sulci of the brain.

The final line of anatomical protection of the brain from external forces comes from the ventricles within the brain. There are 4 cavities within the brain that arise from expansions of the central canal of the spinal cord. The cavities are called ventricles. The ventricles protect the brain by absorbing external forces through the displacement of CSF throughout the cavities.[7] The CSF fills the 4 ventricles of the brain and surrounds the outer surface of the brain and spinal cord, creating a floating cushion of fluid that functions to absorb shock.

Injury Mechanisms

Typically, the mechanism of injury (MOI) in sports medicine is identified by simply asking the athlete what happened. However, in regard to SRCs, this simple question is insufficient to formulate even a preliminary construct of the MOI. In order for the sports emergency care team to know the nature of the MOI associated with a SRC, the sports medicine professional must identify whether the injury was a coup or contra-coup type and whether the injury resulted from focal or diffuse trauma. The type of injury and the type of trauma are biomechanical factors that provide a complete picture of the MOI and can be used to steer the remainder of the clinical assessment.

Cerebral concussions represent the most common brain injury in athletics. These injuries are predominately caused by biomechanical factors. A forceful external blow to a nonmoving head can result in injury to the brain directly beneath the area of the cranium that received the blow. These injuries are referred to as coup injuries, an example being a blow from another player's helmet or a cross check using a hockey or lacrosse stick when the head is not in motion.[3] Another type of injury results from a moving head colliding with a stationary object. These injuries are referred to as contra coup injuries and result in maximal injury on the side of the brain opposite the cranial impact. This may result from an athlete falling down and hitting his or her head on the floor. Both coup and contra-coup injuries may result in intracranial cerebral trauma. By assessing the likelihood of a coup or contra-coup type of injury, the sports medicine professional can better ascertain what lobes of the brain may have been affected by the injury and can develop more sensitive further assessment by asking questions that specifically address the function of those structures most likely affected. This is not to say that all other areas of the CNS are ignored, but that more specific questions can be asked in addition to standard assessment questions.

Once the type of injury has been determined, the type of trauma experienced by the cerebrum should be classified as either focal or diffuse. Focal injuries result from a high-velocity, low-mass force applied to a concentrated area of the cranium. Head injuries that result in death are typically those associated with this focal trauma. Examples of focal trauma include being struck by a baseball, hockey puck, lacrosse ball, or golf ball. Diffuse injuries result from trauma caused by a low-velocity, high-mass blow resulting in a force that is directed over a larger area of the brain.[8,9] Diffuse trauma may be exemplified by a helmeted athlete being struck about the helmet. The nature of protective athletic helmets is to diffuse trauma by spreading it out over the entire shell of the helmet such that no one particular area of the head receives the trauma. The sports emergency care team, upon determining the type of injury and the type of trauma, has a complete understanding of the mechanism of injury, which will provide vital information that can be compared to various signs and symptoms pertaining to acute conditions resulting from SRC. The comparisons between the MOI and various acute signs and symptoms of possible life-threatening conditions allow the sports emergency care team to conduct a more sensitive clinical assessment that may result in uncovering subtle signs and symptoms of life-threatening epidural and subdural hematoma and second impact syndrome (SIS).

Acute Effects of Sports-Related Concussion

Epidural hematoma usually results from a focal blow to the temporal area of the cranium with a significant chance for simultaneous fracture of the temporal bone. Fracture of the temporal bone may encroach on the middle meningeal groove, leading to disruption of the middle meningeal artery and rapid bleeding that quickly increases intracranial pressure. Intracranial bleeding separates the dura mater from the inside of the skull, creating a medical emergency requiring neurosurgery. Epidural hematoma may present with a brief period of unconsciousness followed by a period of consciousness before the athlete enters a coma. An example of an epidural hematoma is an athlete who has been struck with a projectile object such as a baseball. The athlete may be stunned or may momentarily lose consciousness. The athlete may complain of a severe headache upon regaining full consciousness within a few minutes. The athlete begins a downward progression of deteriorating consciousness within a short period of time following regaining full consciousness, leading to stupor before finally falling into a coma within 15 min to 20 min. Epidural hematoma is a life-threatening condition that may result in death within 15 min to 30 min.

Subdural hematoma is also a life-threatening complication of trauma to the brain that is a medical emergency. In most instances of subdural hematoma, an athlete loses consciousness and remains unconscious. On occasion, an athlete suffering a subdural hematoma may regain consciousness and be able to walk off the field under his or her own power; however, he or she may soon collapse due to rapid bleeding and associated swelling of the brain. Subdural hematoma may develop over a period of time. The signs and symptoms of subdural hematoma may not be readily observable at the time of injury and acute assessment. Therefore, it is important to observe the athlete closely over a 24-hour period. If signs and symptoms of postconcussion syndrome persist, the athlete should be referred for further medical assessment.

There are many overlapping signs and symptoms between epidural and subdural hematoma that make it nearly impossible for sports emergency care personnel conducting an acute assessment to make any accurate distinction between them. However, one sign of significance that sports emergency care personnel must be attuned to and specifically assess for is the lucid interval. An athlete suffering a lucid interval will present with a period of lost or altered consciousness followed by a period during which it appears the athlete has recovered. Shortly after the apparent recovery period, an athlete suffering a lucid interval will, again, present with signs and symptoms related to a concussion that may rapidly deteriorate. Although the lucid interval cannot be used to distinguish between an epidural and subdural hematoma, it is a significant indicator of some type of hematoma or other condition that is causing an increase in intracranial pressure that is a medical emergency, indicating the need for immediate transport of the athlete to the nearest emergency room.[10]

Athletes who are allowed to return to competition prior to the complete resolution of all post-traumatic symptoms are at risk of a relatively minor yet fatal second blow, referred to as SIS. It has been theorized that SIS causes the autoregulatory centers of the brain to break down, resulting in uncontrollable cerebral edema. The uncontrollable edema resulting from SIS can lead to outward signs and symptoms involving the cranial nerves within a matter of minutes, and in 50% of all cases, results in catastrophic consequences, as the onset of the condition is virtually impossible to control. SIS is rare, but it has been linked to deaths in athletics since it was first widely described in the early

1980s.[2,10-12] Acute signs and symptoms of an athlete suffering from SIS may resemble a simple concussion; however, the stunned athlete will rapidly lose consciousness and fall into a coma.[11] Cranial nerve pressure resulting from cerebral edema results in dilating pupils that are unresponsive to light. Pressure builds as the swelling continues, and the athlete will begin to show signs of respiratory distress and loss of coordination and motor control.[10]

Medical emergencies such as epidural and subdural hematoma and SIS are certainly conditions that sports emergency care personnel must account for during clinical assessment. However, the more likely acute result of a SRC is the onset of a metabolic cellular cascade that may be responsible for the acute and chronic nature of most SRCs.[3] Cells within the brain suffer acute effects resulting from trauma to the brain that may last for a brief period of a few seconds or minutes or may last for 10 days or more. The acute metabolic changes within a cell may result in spreading depression or the rapid and successive depolarization of adjacent cells within a wide area of the brain. Spreading depression may result in acute loss of consciousness, amnesia, and cognitive impairment. After all the effected cells have been repolarized, all signs and symptoms associated with spreading depression may be completely resolved. However, it is likely that there will be lingering cellular effects that may delay recovery for up to 10 days or more.[13]

Assessment Strategy: The Progressive Algorithm for Assessment of Sports-Related Concussion

During acute assessment of SRC, sports emergency care personnel do not have the opportunity to conduct and assess the most objective measures of the onset of a metabolic cascade, hematoma, or second impact syndrome that are available during postacute assessment. Therefore, sports emergency care personnel must rely on effective observation of the subtle signs and symptoms resulting from a possible SRC to make decisions regarding proper acute management. Effective observation of the subtle signs and symptoms of a SRC requires a thorough and sensitive clinical assessment to ensure that the onset of subtle signs and symptoms indicating the need for immediate transport to a regional emergency room or physician is not overlooked. The Progressive Algorithm for Assessment of Sports-Related Concussion (PASRC) is an acute assessment strategy that provides an organized approach to acute assessment of SRC to minimize the chances of overlooking subtle signs and symptoms and provides a means for making acute management decisions regarding the need for immediate transport to the nearest emergency room or physician referral. The PASRC is detailed in Figure 8-1.

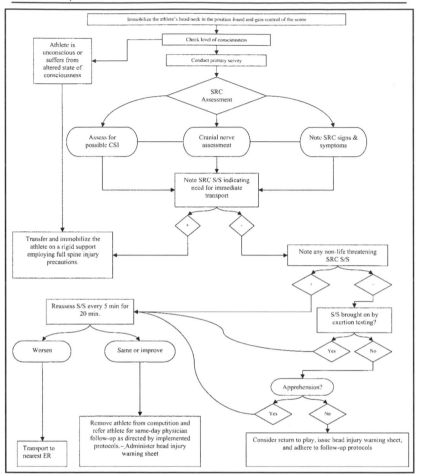

Figure 8-1. Progressive algorithm for the assessment of SRC. (© Sports Medicine Concepts. Reproduced with permission.)

The PASRC, like all other acute sports injury assessments, is preceded by gaining control of the scene and conducting a primary injury survey. It is good practice in athletics to initiate control of the scene by first gaining control of the athlete. Gaining control of the athlete reduces the risk of secondary injury due to unnecessary movement. Gaining control of an injured athlete should be done immediately by placing one hand on the sternum or back, depending on the position of the athlete, and using the other hand to stabilize the athlete's head and neck. Upon determining a mechanism of injury indicating the possibility of a SRC, the sports emergency care team should initiate more formal immobilization of the head and neck using both hands to immobilize the head and neck to the torso while completing the remainder of the PASRC.

The PASRC includes 3 critical assessment categories that serve as failsafe "fuses." If certain signs and symptoms are observed within any of the 3 critical stages of the assessment, the failsafe fuse is blown and the sports medicine team activates EMS to aid in caring for and transporting the athlete. Once a fuse is blown in the PASRC and EMS is activated, the assessment for the purpose of determining the need to transport the athlete is over. The initial caregivers maintain vital signs while waiting for EMS team members to arrive. Together, the sports emergency care team conducts necessary ongoing assessment during transfer of the athlete to a rigid support, immobilization, and transport of the athlete to the nearest emergency room. After the PASRC indicates the need for transport, unnecessary assessment should be avoided because it increases the likelihood of extraneous movement of the athlete, delays transport, and provides an opportunity for apparent improvements in signs and symptoms, causing the sports emergency care team to mistakenly reverse a critical decision to transport.

The first critical assessment category in the PASRC involves ruling out the possibility of concurrent injury to the cervical spine. Because the MOI for SRC and CSI can be very similar, the athlete must be specifically assessed for indicators of injury to the cervical spine. If the athlete presents with signs and symptoms that indicate the possibility of CSI, the athlete must be transferred to a rigid support and transported to the nearest emergency room using full spine injury precautions. The presence of a SRC can complicate assessment of possible CSI because the mental status and level of consciousness may interfere with the athlete's ability to understand and respond appropriately to the sports emergency care team's questions. An inability of the athlete to understand and respond to the sports emergency care team's questions pertaining to concurrent CSI is a critical failsafe fuse. If the team cannot definitively rule out the possibility of CSI, it must be assumed that a CSI exists, and the athlete must be transported using full spine injury precautions.

The second critical assessment category in the PASRC involves assessment of the athlete's cranial nerves. The cranial nerves are part of the peripheral nervous system, but they are particularly vulnerable to complications resulting from intracranial pressure because of their location at the base of the brain. Thus, assessment of the cranial nerves can provide early clues indicating the presence of increased intracranial pressure. Additionally, a thoughtful review of the motor and sensory functions of the cranial nerves reveals that many of the basic questions asked by sports emergency care personnel during assessment of a possible concussion are actually assessments of the motor or sensory function of 1 of the 12 cranial nerves. Therefore, a comprehensive assessment of the 12 cranial nerves provides the foundation for a very organized and thorough battery of questions pertaining to the presence of a SRC. Table 8-1

Table 8-1

CRANIAL NERVE ASSESSMENT GUIDE

Nerve	Name	Function	Test for
I	Olfactory	Smell	Have the athlete identify odors with each nostril (eg, analgesic cream, antiseptic).
II	Optic	Visual acuity	Have the athlete identify number of fingers or figures on flashcards.
		Visual field	Approach the athlete's eyes from the side using your finger or pen light.
III	Oculomotor	Pupillary reaction	Check pupillary reaction in each eye using a pen light.
IV	Trochlear	Eye movements	Have the athlete follow a pen light without moving his or her head.
V	Trigeminal	Facial sensation	Have the athlete identify the areas of the face that are being touched.
		Motor	Have the athlete hold his or mouth open against resistance.
VI	Abducens	Motor	Check the athlete's lateral eye movements.
VII	Facial	Motor	Have the athlete smile, wrinkle forehead, frown, puff cheeks, and wink each eye.
		Sensory	Have the athlete identify familiar tastes (sports drink, toothpaste, etc).
VIII	Acoustic	Hearing	Have the athlete identify sounds in both ears (tuning fork, snapping fingers).
		Balance	Check the athlete's balance (Rhomberg sign).

(continued)

Table 8-1 (continued)

CRANIAL NERVE ASSESSMENT GUIDE

Nerve	Name	Function	Test for
IX	Glossopharyngeal	Swallowing	Have the athlete say "ah" and swallow hard.
X	Vagus	Gag reflex	Test the gag reflex (tongue depressor).
XI	Spinal	Neck strength	Have the athlete complete full active range of motion (AROM), shoulder shrugs against resistance.
XII	Hypoglossal	Tongue movement and strength	Have the athlete stick out his or her tongue and move it around. Apply resistance with a tongue depressor or a finger wrapped with gauze.

© Sport Medicine Concepts. Reproduced with permission.

provides an overview of the motor and sensory functions associated with the 12 cranial nerves as well as a specific acute test that can be easily administered.

The final critical assessment category in the PASRC involves the sports emergency care team assessing for the following signs and symptoms of SRC that are not observed during assessment of the 12 cranial nerves[3]:

- Dizziness
- Drowsiness
- Excessive sleepiness
- Easily distracted
- Fatigue
- Feel "in a fog"
- Feel "slowed down"
- Headache
- Inappropriate emotions
- Irritability
- Loss of consciousness

- Loss of orientation
- Memory deficits
- Nausea
- Anxiety
- Personality changes
- Seeing stars
- Photophobia
- Sensitivity to noise
- Vomiting
- Vacant stare/glassy eyes

Upon completion of the 3 critical assessment categories in the PASRC, the sports emergency care team must determine if any of the signs and symptoms observed indicate the need for immediate transfer, immobilization, and transport of the athlete to the nearest emergency room. Signs and symptoms indicating the need for immediate transport to the nearest emergency room include the following[3]:

- Indications of CSI
- Lucid interval
- Worsening neurological function
- Decreasing loss of consciousness
- Decreased or irregular respiration or pulse
- Pupils that are unequal, dilated, or unreactive to light
- Signs and symptoms of skull fracture
- Seizure activity
- Acute cranial nerve deficits
- Mental status changes

If there are no signs and symptoms indicating the need for immediate transport of the athlete, the sports emergency care team should assess the athlete at rest for any non–life-threatening signs and symptoms of SRC by bringing the athlete to the sideline and recording all signs and symptoms every 5 min for 20 min.[3] The athlete should be monitored for deteriorating or worsening signs and symptoms during the 20-min sideline observation. If the athlete's signs and symptoms deteriorate during the 20-min sideline observation, EMS should be activated to transport the athlete to the nearest emergency room. Figure 8-2 provides a sample checklist to record signs and symptoms of SRC over a 20-min period.

If the athlete's signs and symptoms remain consistent or improve throughout the 20-min sideline observation, the athlete should be kept from competition and referred to a sports physician for same-day follow-up. In

Acute Concussion Signs and Symptoms Record for

_____

Date : _____

Instructions: At each time interval indicate the status of existing concussion signs and symptoms by marking an (I) if the sign or symptom improved, a (W) if the S/S worsened, or a (N) if there was no change from the prior interval.

* Pupils equal and reactive to light

SRC Signs and Symptoms	Time of Injury	5 min follow-up	10 min follow-up	15 min follow-up	20 min follow-up
Neck pain					
Amnesia					
Dizziness					
Headache					
Nausea					
Feel "in a fog"					
Vision					
PEARL*					
Drowsiness					
Easily distracted					
Over emotional					
Irritability					
Loss of orientation					
Memory deficits					
Anxiety					
Balance abnormalities					
Personality changes					
Tinnitis					
Seeing stars					
Photophobia					
Sensitivity to noise					
Vacant stare					
Comments:					

Figure 8-2. Sample checklist for signs and symptoms of concussion. (© Sports Medicine Concepts. Reproduced with permission.)

addition to referring the athlete to a sports physician, a head injury warning sheet should be reviewed with the athlete, the athlete's parents or guardian, and the coach. A head injury warning sheet is a written set of signs and symptoms that can be used to monitor the athlete when he or she is not being observed by sports emergency care personnel. The head injury warning sheet should also include instructions for the athlete to follow in the event that any

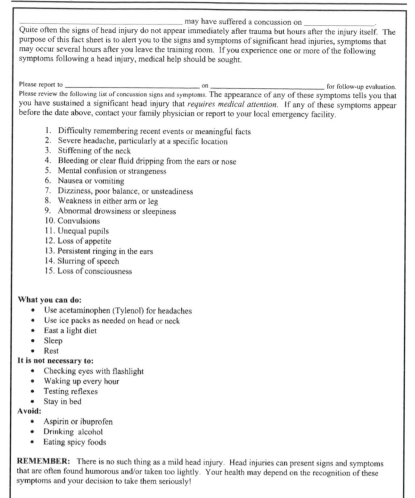

_____ may have suffered a concussion on _____.
Quite often the signs of head injury do not appear immediately after trauma but hours after the injury itself. The purpose of this fact sheet is to alert you to the signs and symptoms of significant head injuries, symptoms that may occur several hours after you leave the training room. If you experience one or more of the following symptoms following a head injury, medical help should be sought.

Please report to _____ on _____ for follow-up evaluation.
Please review the following list of concussion signs and symptoms. The appearance of any of these symptoms tells you that you have sustained a significant head injury that *requires medical attention*. If any of these symptoms appear before the date above, contact your family physician or report to your local emergency facility.

1. Difficulty remembering recent events or meaningful facts
2. Severe headache, particularly at a specific location
3. Stiffening of the neck
4. Bleeding or clear fluid dripping from the ears or nose
5. Mental confusion or strangeness
6. Nausea or vomiting
7. Dizziness, poor balance, or unsteadiness
8. Weakness in either arm or leg
9. Abnormal drowsiness or sleepiness
10. Convulsions
11. Unequal pupils
12. Loss of appetite
13. Persistent ringing in the ears
14. Slurring of speech
15. Loss of consciousness

What you can do:
- Use acetaminophen (Tylenol) for headaches
- Use ice packs as needed on head or neck
- East a light diet
- Sleep
- Rest

It is not necessary to:
- Checking eyes with flashlight
- Waking up every hour
- Testing reflexes
- Stay in bed

Avoid:
- Aspirin or ibuprofen
- Drinking alcohol
- Eating spicy foods

REMEMBER: There is no such thing as a mild head injury. Head injuries can present signs and symptoms that are often found humorous and/or taken too lightly. Your health may depend on the recognition of these symptoms and your decision to take them seriously!

Figure 8-3. Sample head injury warning sheet. (© Sports Medicine Concepts. Reproduced with permission.)

signs and symptoms indicated on the head injury warning sheet are observed. Figure 8-3 provides and example of a head injury warning sheet.

If no signs or symptoms of SRC are observed while the athlete is at rest, the athlete should be re-examined after completing a series of exertional maneuvers such as jogging, biking, sit-ups, or push-ups.[3] If life-threatening signs and symptoms arise as a result of the exertional maneuvers, EMS should be activated to transport the athlete to the nearest emergency room. If exertional maneuvers bring about non–life-threatening signs and symptoms, the athlete should be removed from competition and assessed at 5-min intervals for the next 20 min to observe for the onset of signs and symptoms indicating the need to transport the athlete to the nearest emergency room. If no life-threatening signs and symptoms emerge after 20 min, the athlete should be referred to a sports physician for same-day follow-up.

Should exertional maneuvers fail to bring about signs and symptoms, the sports emergency care team should inquire about any apprehension that the athlete may have with regard to returning to competition. If neither the athlete nor the sports emergency care personnel is apprehensive about returning the athlete to competition, return to play may be considered in accordance with implemented protocols. In addition, the athlete should be monitored throughout the remainder of the game to ensure that delayed signs and symptoms do not emerge. Finally, regardless of the athlete's apparent condition following same-day return to play, a head injury warning sheet should be administered to the athlete, parents, and any others that will be in a position to observe the athlete for any length of time before returning for follow-up care.

The acute sideline assessment of SRC provides an opportunity for sports emergency care personnel to perform a few simple, but very effective objective assessments that may demonstrate the existence of SRC signs and symptoms when subjective measures fail to do so. A simple sideline test to assess postural sway, indicative of balance abnormalities, is the Balance Error Scoring System (BESS) conducted on a foam surface.[3] To administer the BESS on the sideline, have the athlete perform a double-leg stance followed by a single-leg stance and tandem stance, each for 20 seconds using the nondominant leg. During each test, the subject should be instructed to assume the required stance, place his or her hands on his or her hips, and close his or her eyes. The BESS score is then calculated by adding 1 error point for each of the following:

- Lifting hands off hips
- Opening eyes
- Stepping, stumbling, or falling
- Moving the hip into more than 30 degrees of flexion or abduction
- Lifting the forefoot or heel
- Remaining out of the testing position for more than 5 seconds

Upon completion of the BESS test, document the score on the SRC Signs and Symptoms Record to trend results over time and for future comparison. The BESS test has been found to be most effective when used to compare performance following a concussion to the athlete's baseline measure.[14,15] However, normative data that can be use to interpret BESS scores do exist.[3]

Neuropsychological testing is gaining acceptance as a standard of care in SRC management.[16-20] Neuropsychological tests have been shown to measure subtle differences in the information processing speed of athletes having suffered a concussion versus those who had not.[3,18,19] Neuropsychological tests offer sports emergency care teams a number of promising benefits, including the ability to identify individual differences in pre-season status to help physicians accurately gauge the effects of an injury, providing early evidence of postconcussion symptoms, unmasking players' attempts to hide symptoms, tracking injury status, aiding return-to-play decision making, reducing the risk of second impact syndrome, and helping to determine the long-term impact of multiple concussions.[2,16,17,19]

A simple acute neuropsychological test that should be considered for use in acute sideline assessment of sports-related concussion is the standardized assessment of concussion test (SAC).[18,19] The SAC test is divided into 4 assessment categories: orientation, immediate memory recall, concentration, and delayed recall. The athlete's orientation is assessed by asking the athlete the month, date, day of the week, year, and time (within 1 hour). When the athlete correctly answers each of the orientation questions, one point is given. The total orientation score is then calculated as the total correct answer points out of a possible score of 5.

Sample SAC Orientation Test		
Month	0	1
Date	0	1
Day of Week	0	1
Year	0	1
Time (within 1 hr)	0	1
Orientation Total Score	___ /5	

Next, immediate recall is assessed by asking the athlete to repeat a list of 5 words over 3 different trials. Three individual trials are conducted beginning with the examiner listing the five same words. The athlete is then asked to repeat the list in any order to complete each trial. All 3 trails are completed regardless of the score on any previous trial. The total immediate recall score is calculated by adding the number of words the athlete is able to recall over all 3 trials out of a possible total score of 15.

Sample SAC Immediate Recall Test						
List	Trial 1		Trial 2		Trial 3	
Elbow	0	1	0	1	0	1
Apple	0	1	0	1	0	1
Carpet	0	1	0	1	0	1
Saddle	0	1	0	1	0	
Total score	___ /15					

The athlete's concentration is assessed next by asking the athlete to list, in reverse order, a series of digits verbally given by the examiner. The SAC involves 4 different strings of numbers. The examiner should ask the athlete to repeat the first string in reverse order. If the athlete is not able to repeat the list in reverse order, he or she is given another chance. If the athlete is able to repeat the number string correctly after trial 1 or 2, the next string length is given to the athlete. If the athlete is not able to correctly repeat the string length after the second attempt, the test is concluded. One point is provided for each correct string length. During the concentration test, the athlete is also asked to repeat the months in reverse order. One point is provided when the athlete is able to repeat all 12 months in reverse order. The total concentration score is out of a possible 5.

Sample SAC Concentration Test			
Digits in reverse order			
4-9-3	6-2-9	0	1
3-8-1-4	3-2-7-9	0	1
6-2-9-7-1	1-5-2-8-6	0	1
7-1-8-4-6-2	5-3-9-1-4-8	0	1
Months in reverse order		0	1
Total Concentration Score	____ /5		

Finally, the SAC assesses delayed recall by asking the athlete to repeat the prior list of words given during the immediate memory test. A point is provided for each word the athlete is able to recall in any order. The delayed recall score is out of a total of 5 possible points.

Sample SAC Delayed Recall Test		
Elbow	0	1
Apple	0	1
Carpet	0	1
Saddle	0	1
Bubble	0	1
Total Delayed Recall Score	____ /5	

Upon completion of all 4 SAC categories, the total SAC score is calculated by adding each of the categories for an overall score out of a possible 30 points. The SAC score can then be used for comparison to normative data, but the preferred method of assessment is to compare the SAC score to baseline scores. The SAC test comes in 3 forms that can be administered at various stages for tracking injury recovery, making return-to-play decisions, and assessing extent of injury. The SAC tests have been found to be most effective when administered as part of the pre-participation examination to test the athlete's cognitive status before the season, then within 24 hours after the injury, and within 5 days after the injury episode.[18,19]

Sample SAC Score Summary	
Orientation	___ /5
Immediate Recall	___ /15
Concentration	___ /5
Delayed Recall	___ /5
Overall Score	___ /30

When incorporated into a total management plan including a sports medicine team approach and implementation of accepted protocols, it appears that neuropsychological testing is an effective means for the sports medicine team to uncover subtle signs and symptoms of head injury that might escape traditional tests. Recognition of these important signs and symptoms can help sports emergency care personnel determine if an athlete has suffered a concussion, classify the extent of injury, and make prudent acute management.

Historically, SRCs have been identified, classified, and managed based on a number of head injury grading scales, though none have been universally accepted. The 2 most recognized in sports medicine are detailed in Tables 8-2 and 8-3.[21-23] Classifying the extent of injury using grading scales requires that some signs and symptoms be tracked for hours, days, or complete resolution. Acute or emergency care of SRC obviously does not provide sufficient time to track signs and symptoms in order to assign an appropriate grade. In addition, criteria for determining the most appropriate acute management of an athlete who has suffered a SRC is completely independent of any classification and is completely dependent on the athlete's present symptomatology. Therefore, the use of grading scales and the determination of the corresponding grade of injury is of little practical use during the emergency care and management of SRC, particularly when determining the need for immediate transport or same-day physician referral. It may be that grading scales are most useful in determining the grade of an athlete's injury after all signs and symptoms have resolved as a record for comparison with any future SRC the athlete may suffer.

Though there is no consensus regarding the classification of brain injuries based on signs and symptoms, it is very much agreed upon that an athlete who suffers signs or symptoms of a concussion should not be permitted to return

Table 8-2

AMERICAN ACADEMY OF NEUROLOGY CONCUSSION GRADING SCALE

Grade 1 (mild)	Transient confusion; no LOC*; symptoms and mental status abnormalities resolve in <15 min
Grade 2 (moderate)	Transient confusion; no LOC; symptoms and mental status abnormalities last >15 min
Grade 3 (severe)	Any LOC

* LOC indicates loss of consciousness.

Table 8-3

CANTU EVIDENCE-BASED GRADING SYSTEM FOR CONCUSSION

Grade 1 (mild)	No LOC*, PTA† <30 min, PCSS‡ <24 hours
Grade 2 (moderate)	LOC <1 min or PTA ≥30 min ≤24 hours or PCSS ≥24 hours ≤7 days
Grade 3 (severe)	LOC ≥1 min or PTA ≥24 hours or PCSS ≥7 days

* LOC indicates loss of consciousness
† PTA indicates post-traumatic amnesia (anterograde/retrograde)
‡ PCSS indicates postconcussion signs and symptoms other than amnesia

to competition.[2,23,24] Lingering signs and symptoms of concussion indicate that the metabolic cellular cascade outlined earlier has not completely resolved and would predispose the athlete to recurrent and more severe injuries such as second impact syndrome and postconcussion syndrome.

Conclusion

Acute assessment of SRC requires a thorough and organized approach to ensure that the subtle signs and symptoms indicating the need for emergent transport to the nearest emergency room are not overlooked. The acute assessment of SRC is complicated by the fact that SRC is often associated with delayed onset of symptoms indicative of an underlying life-threatening condition. Therefore, the sports emergency care team must be thorough in assessing the immediate need for transport of the athlete, but must also continue to monitor non–life-threatening signs and symptoms of concussion in order to make prudent decisions regarding the need for further medical follow-up. Further medical follow-up may consist of neuroimaging techniques, neuropsychological testing, and the use of various other concussion assessment tools to aid the sports medicine team in evaluating and making return-to-play decisions.

The process of caring for an athlete who has suffered a SRC can be frustrating for all involved. However, the process must be completed in order to protect the athlete from life-threatening conditions and a possible lifetime of varying degrees of disability resulting from return to play before the athlete has fully recovered.

References

1. Swenson EJ, McKeag DB. Minor head injury evaluation: current state-of-the-art results of survey completed by the American Medical Society for Sports Medicine membership in 1994. Results presented at: Annual meeting of the American Medical Society for Sports Medicine; June 9, 1996; Orlando, Fla.

2. Macciocchi S, Barth JT, Alves W. Neuropsychological functioning and recovery after mild head injury in collegiate athletes. *Neurosurgery.* 1996;39:510-514.

3. Guskiewicz KM, Bruce SL, Cantu RC, et al. National Athletic Trainers' Association position statement: management of sports-related concussion. *Journal of Athletic Training.* 2004;39:280-297.

4. Ogilivie BC, Howe M. Career crisis in sport. *Proceedings of the Fifth World Congress of Sports Psychology.* 1987;3:32-39.

5. Dietzel P. There is life after football. In: LeUness AD, Nation JR, eds. *Sports Psychology: An Introduction.* Chicago, Ill: Nelson-Hall; 1983:436-438.

6. Gray H. The nervous system. In: Pick TP, ed. *Gray's Anatomy.* Philadelphia: Lea & Febiger; 1977.

7. Hollinshead WH, Rosse C. The cranial part of the central nervous system. In: *Textbook of Anatomy.* 5th ed. Philadelphia: Harper and Row; 1985.

8. Arnheim DD, Prentice WE. The head and face. In: *Principles of Athletic Training.* 11th ed. St. Louis, Mo: Mosby; 2002.

9. Booher JM, Thibodeau GA. Head and face injuries. In: *Athletic Injury Assessment.* 3rd ed. St. Louis, Mo: Mosby; 1994.

10. Onate JA, Guskiewicz KM, McCrea MA. A comparison of concussion incidence and recovery in college football players with and without previous history of concussion. [Abstract]. *Journal of Athletic Training.* 2000;35(2):S54.

11. Centers for Disease Control and Prevention. Sports-related recurrent brain injuries: United States. *MMWR.* 1997;46(NM10):224-227.

12. Shell D, Carico G, Patton RM. Can subdural hematoma result from repeated minor head injury? *Phys Sports Med.* 1993;21:74-84.

13. Giza CC, Hovda DA. Ionic and metabolic consequences of concussion. In: Cantu RC, ed. *Neurological Athletic Head and Spine Injuries.* Philadelphia: WB Saunders Company; 2000:80-100.

14. Lovell MR, Collins MW, Iverson GL, et al. Recovery from mild concussion in high school athletes. *J Neurosurg.* 2003;98:296-301.

15. Guskiewicz KM, Cantu RC. The concussion puzzle: evaluation of sports-related concussion. *Am J Sports Med.* 2004;6:13-21.

16. Kelly JP, Rosenberg JH. Practice parameters: the management of concussion in sports summary statement. *Neurology.* 1997;48:581-585.

17. Lovell MR, Collins MW. Neuropsychological assessment of the college football player. *J Head Traum Rehab.* 1998;12:9-26.

18. McCrea M, Kelly JP, Kluge J, Ackley B, Randolph C. Standardized assessment of concussion in football players. *Neurology.* 1998;48:586-588.

19. McCrea M, Kelly JP, Randolph C, et al. Standardized assessment of concussion (SAC): onsite mental evaluation of the athlete. *J Head Trauma Rehabil.* 1998;13:27-35.

20. Bleiberg J, Cernich AN, Cameron K, et al. Duration of cognitive impairment after sports concussion. *Neurosurgery.* 2004;54:1073-1080.

21. Practice parameter: the management of concussion in sports (summary statement). Report of the Quality Standards Subcommittee of the American Academy of Neurology. *Neurology.* 1997;48:581-585.

22. Cantu RC. Posttraumatic retrograde and anterograde amnesia: pathophysiology and implications in grading and safe return to play. *Journal of Athletic Training.* 2001;36:244-248.

23. Cantu RC. Guidelines for return to contact sports after cerebral concussion. *Phys Sports Med.* 1986;14:75-83.

24. Kelly JP, Rosenberg JH. Diagnosis and management of concussion in sports. *Neurology.* 1997;48:575-580.

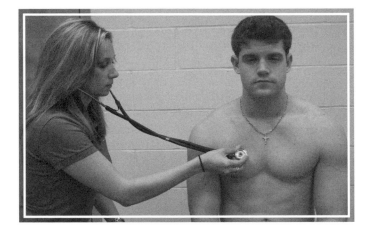

Chapter 9 — Injuries to the Thoracic Region

Michael Prybicien, MA, ATC, EMT-B, CSCS

Acute thoracic injuries can be among the most serious in sports because they can impose a threat of long-term disability and in the most severe cases even death. They have the potential to be catastrophic in nature because they can affect the spinal cord; nerves around the spinal cord (which are responsible for motor and sensory activity); and even the heart, lungs, and various other organs. Fortunately, thoracic injuries are usually nonemergency acute conditions such as sprains, strains, and contusions.

Review of Clinically Relevant Anatomy

The thorax (Figure 9-1) is a bone cavity that is formed by 12 pairs of ribs that join posteriorly with the thoracic spine and anteriorly with the sternum. The intercostal neurovascular bundle runs along the inferior surface of each rib. The inner side of the thoracic cavity and the lung itself are lined with a thin layer of tissue called the pleura. The space between the 2 pleural layers is normally only a potential space. However, this space may be occupied by air, forming a pneumothorax, or blood, forming a hemothorax. This potential space can hold 3 L of fluid on each side in an adult.

One lung occupies each thorax cavity. The mediastinum is between the chest cavity and contains the heart, aorta, superior and inferior vena cava, trachea, major bronchi, and esophagus. The spinal cord is protected by the vertebral column. The diaphragm separates the thoracic organs from the abdominal cavity. The upper abdominal organs, including the spleen, liver, kidneys, pancreas, and stomach, are protected by the lower rib cage. Any patient with a penetrating thoracic wound (ie, javelin) at the level of the nipples or lower should be assumed to have an abdominal injury as well as a thoracic injury. Similarly, blunt deceleration injuries such as direct blows from

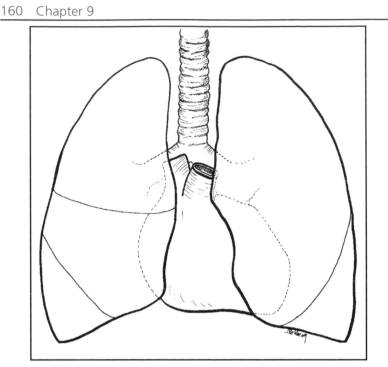

Figure 9-1. Anterior view of the thorax. (Illustration by Joelle Rehberg, DO.)

a helmet or other body parts can often injure both the thoracic and abdominal structures.

The thoracic spine consists of 12 vertical columns (vertebrae) connected by "facet joints." A disc with a lining and a center filled with a gelatinous substance lies between each of these vertebrae. These discs act as shock absorbers and provide the spinal column with its flexibility. When an athlete runs and jumps, these discs absorb the impact as well as prevent the vertebrae from grinding against one another.

Four muscle groups, the abdominals, the extensors, and 2 sets of paraspinal muscles, control the thoracic spinal column. Within the spinal cord is a massive trunk of nerves that runs down the length of the spinal column from the brain to the sacrum. Smaller nerves branch out from the main trunk at each vertebra. These nerves travel to the arms, torso, and the legs. The brain can send out electrical impulses through these nerves to the various tissues to make them function. The brain can also receive feedback from the tissues through these nerves.

Evaluation and Assessment

When evaluating an athlete with a possible thoracic injury, sports emergency care providers should always assume the worse because it is extremely important that potential life-threatening injuries are not overlooked. During the initial evaluation, search first for the most serious injuries. As with any athletic injury, the mechanism of injury is extremely important in caring for the most severe thoracic injuries. Thoracic injuries may be the result of blunt or penetrating trauma. Blunt trauma, which can occur in most contact sports, can result in a force being distributed over a large area, and visceral injuries occur from deceleration, shearing forces, compression, or bursting. Penetrating injuries, which are less common, can occur from objects that are inadvertently on the field or court surface or objects that are airborne such as a javelin. The distribution of forces is typically over a much smaller area in penetrating injuries.

Oftentimes, thoracic injury results in tissue hypoxia. Tissue hypoxia may result from the following:

- Inadequate oxygen delivery to the tissues secondary to airway obstruction
- Hypovolemia from blood loss
- Asymmetrical lung expansion
- Changes in pleural pressures from tension pneumothorax
- Pump failure from severe myocardial injury

The major symptoms of chest injury include shortness of breath, chest pain, and respiratory distress. The signs indicative of chest injury include shock, hemoptysis, cyanosis, chest wall contusion, flail chest, open wounds, distended neck veins, tracheal deviation, or subcutaneous emphysema. Check the lungs for the presence, quality, and equality of breath sounds. Life-threatening, sports-related thoracic injuries should be identified immediately. Some sports-related thoracic injuries will be detected during the primary survey while others may not be detected until a more detailed examination is conducted.

The following injuries are detected during the primary survey:

- Airway obstruction
- Tension/traumatic pneumothorax
- Spontaneous pneumothorax
- Massive hemothorax
- Flail chest
- Cardiac tamponade

The following injuries are more likely to be detected during the detailed examination:

- Traumatic aorta rupture
- Tracheal or bronchial tree injury
- Myocardial contusion
- Diaphragmatic tear
- Esophageal injury
- Pulmonary contusion
- Sternal fractures or contusion
- Rib fractures or contusions
- Costochondral separation/dislocation
- Thoracic spine fracture/contusions
- Thoracic muscle strains

AIRWAY OBSTRUCTION

Airway obstruction recognition is vital. Airway management is a challenge that must be met in the care of the life-threatening sports injury. Refer to Chapter 4 for additional information on management of airway and breathing emergencies. Finally, always assume a spinal injury in the unconscious down athlete when securing the airway.

TENSION/TRAUMATIC PNEUMOTHORAX

This injury can occur when a one-way valve is created from either blunt or penetrating trauma. Air can enter but cannot leave the pleural space. This causes an increase in the intrathoracic pressure, which will collapse the lung and increase pressure on the mediastinum. This pressure will eventually collapse the superior and inferior vena cava, resulting in a loss of venous return to the heart. A shift of the trachea and mediastinum away from the side of the tension pneumothorax will also compromise ventilation of the other lung, although this is a late phenomenon.

Clinical signs of a tension pneumothorax (Figure 9-2) include apprehension, agitation, cyanosis, diminished breath sounds and hyperresonance to percussion on the affected side, cold clammy skin, distended neck veins, and hypotension. Tracheal deviation, or a shifting of the trachea toward the side of the functioning lung, is usually a late sign (if at all), and its absence does not rule out a tension pneumothorax.

SPONTANEOUS PNEUMOTHORAX

Spontaneous pneumothorax is a rare condition found occasionally in athletes. This condition can be fatal if not appropriately detected and managed. Diagnosis depends on a thorough understanding of possible presenting signs and symptoms such as chest pain, dyspnea, and diminished breath sounds.

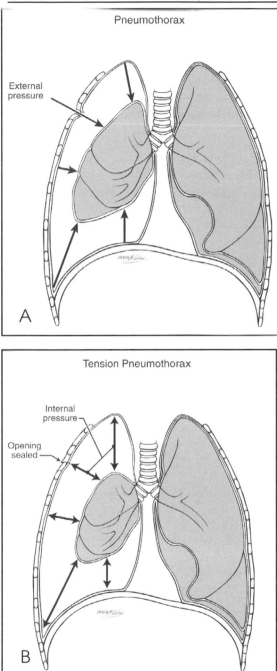

Figure 9-2. Pneumothorax. (Reprinted with permission from O'Connor DP. *Clinical Pathology for Athletic Trainers: Recognizing Systemic Disease.* Thorofare, NJ: SLACK Incorporated; 2001:71.)

Regardless of whether a pneumothorax occurs spontaneously or from trauma, early and accurate diagnosis is essential. The classic complaint of an athlete with a pneumothorax is chest pain. The pain can be vague but is usually localized to the side of the affected lung and can radiate to the shoulder, neck, and/or back. Often pain can be associated with dyspnea on exertion and/or a dry cough. Other classic findings of pneumothorax include tachypnea, tachycardia, hyperresonance to percussion of the affected chest area, diminished breath sounds, and fremitus on the side of the affected lung.

Although the factors that cause or contribute to a spontaneous pneumothorax are not clearly understood, it has been suggested that a family history and a tall, thin body build can be associated factors.

Sports-related spontaneous pneumothorax has been documented in weight lifting, football, and jogging. Most cases of spontaneous pneumothorax, however, are not related to exertion or activity.

Clinical signs of a spontaneous pneumothorax include apprehension, agitation, sharp unilateral chest pain, a history of vigorous coughing, and decreased lung sounds unilaterally.

This patient must be transported rapidly to the hospital (Table 9-1) so chest decompression can be performed. A chest tube will also be necessary upon arrival to the hospital.

MASSIVE HEMOTHORAX

A hemothorax (Figure 9-3) occurs when blood enters the pleural space. A massive hemothorax occurs as a result of at least 1500 cc blood loss into the thoracic cavity. Each thoracic cavity may contain up to 3000 cc of blood. A massive hemothorax is more commonly caused by a penetrating trauma but it can also occur from a blunt trauma. Either mechanism of injury may disrupt a major pulmonary or systemic vessel. As blood accumulates within the pleural space, the lung on the affected side is compressed. If enough blood accumulates, the mediastinum will be shifted away from the hemothorax. The inferior and superior vena cava and the contralateral lung are compressed. Thus, the blood loss is complicated by hypoxemia.

Clinical signs and symptoms of massive hemothorax are produced by both hypovolemia and respiratory compromise. The patient may be hypotensive from blood loss and compression of the heart or great veins. Anxiety, apprehension, and confusion are the results of hypovolemia and hypoxemia. Signs and symptoms of hypovolemic shock may be apparent followed by difficulty breathing. The neck veins are usually flat, breath sounds are decreased or absent on the side of the injury, and chest percussion is dull.

Table 9-1

MANAGEMENT OF SPONTANEOUS AND TENSION PNEUMOTHORAX AND HEMOTHORAX

* Establish an open airway.
* Activate EMS if not on the scene.
* Treat for shock.
* Provide supplemental oxygen (avoid positive pressure ventilation).
* Place in a position of comfort or if lying, with affected side down (this occasionally helps).
* Monitor oxygen saturation with pulse oximeter.
* Rapid transport to hospital.

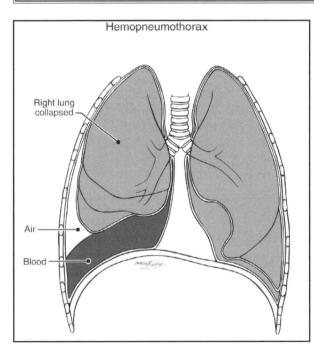

Figure 9-3. Hemothorax. (Reprinted with permission from O'Connor DP. *Clinical Pathology for Athletic Trainers: Recognizing Systemic Disease.* Thorofare, NJ: SLACK Incorporated; 2001:72.)

FLAIL CHEST

Flail chest (Figure 9-4) is defined as a fracture of 2 or more adjacent ribs in at least 2 places. These injuries typically occur in contact sports like football, hockey, wrestling, and lacrosse. In rare cases, they may occur from a severe torsion mechanism in a noncontact sport. The result is a segment of the chest

Figure 9-4. Flail chest. (Illustration by Joelle Rehberg, DO.)

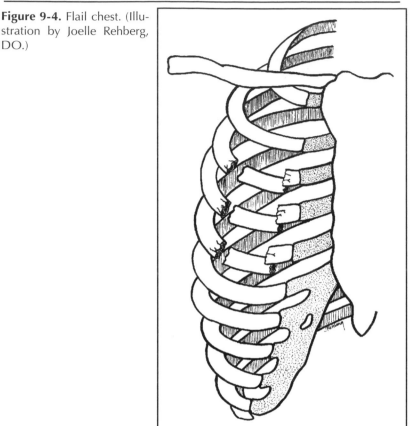

wall that is not in continuity with the thorax. A lateral flail chest or anterior flail chest (sternal separation) may result. With posterior rib fractures, the heavy musculature usually prevents the occurrence of a flail segment. The flail segment moves with paradoxical motion relative to the rest of the chest wall. The force necessary to produce injury also bruises the underlying lung tissue, and the pulmonary contusion can also contribute to hypoxia. The patient is at risk for the development of the other conditions already discussed in this chapter (a hemothorax or pneumothorax). With a large flail segment, the patient may be in marked respiratory distress. Pain from the chest wall injury exacerbates the already impaired respiration from paradoxical motion and the underlying lung contusion. Palpation of the chest may reveal crepitus in addition to the abnormal respiratory movement.

Management of flail chest includes stabilizing the flail segment with manual pressure or a bulky dressing or pillow secured to the chest. Treat for pneumothorax or hemothorax if signs and symptoms are present.

TRACHEAL OR BRONCHIAL TREE INJURY

These injuries are rare in sports because they are usually the result of a penetrating or blunt trauma. The signs and symptoms must be recognized because it can be a fatal condition. This injury is a penetrating upper airway injury that can be associated with major vascular injuries and extensive tissue destruction. Signs and symptoms include shortness of breath, mediastinal shift, subcutaneous emphysema, and hemoptysis. Mechanism of injury and history are vital, and the clinical finding may be subtle. In this blunt injury, either the trachea or mainstream bronchus will be ruptured. The signs that may be present can include subcutaneous emphysema of the chest, face, or neck or even associated pneumothorax or hemothorax.

Management of tracheal or bronchial tree injury includes maintaining an open airway, activating EMS (if not already on scene), administering high-flow supplemental oxygen, and transporting the athlete to the hospital immediately.

DIAPHRAGMATIC TEARS

Tears in the diaphragm may result from a severe blow to the abdomen and can occur in a large variety of sporting events. A sudden increase in intra-abdominal pressure, such as a kick, punch, or elbow to the abdomen, may tear the diaphragm and allow herniation of the abdominal organs into the thoracic cavity. This occurs more commonly on the left side than the right side because the liver protects the right diaphragm. The blunt trauma may produce large radial tears in the diaphragm. Penetrating trauma may also produce holes in the diaphragm, but those tend to be small.

This injury may be difficult to diagnose, even in the hospital. The clinical signs may include the following: marked respiratory distress; diminished breath sounds; and infrequent bowel sounds, which may be heard when the chest is auscultated. The abdomen may present a sucked-in appearance if a large quantity of abdominal contents is in the chest.

Management for diaphragmatic tears includes treating for shock, assisting with breathing, supplemental oxygen, and immediate transfer to a medical facility.

ESOPHAGEAL INJURY

This injury is usually produced by a penetrating trauma, and it is rare in sports. However, sports emergency care personnel must be able to recognize this injury because it can be fatal if unrecognized. Signs and symptoms of esophageal injury include stridor, hoarseness, dysphagia, subcutaneous emphysema, and oropharyngeal/nasopharyngeal bleeding. Management of associated trauma is extremely important as well. Treat for shock, provide supplemental oxygen, and package the patient as soon as possible and transport to a hospital because operative repair will be required for this injury.

PULMONARY CONTUSION

Pulmonary contusion is a common injury that occurs from blunt trauma. Bruising of the lung results from passage of a shock wave through the tissue. Injuries involving high velocity rather than slow crushing are more likely to cause pulmonary contusion. Contusion of the lung may produce marked hypoxemia.

Pulmonary contusions are rarely diagnosed on physical examination. The mechanism of injury may suggest blunt chest trauma, and thus there may be obvious signs of chest wall trauma such as bruising, rib fractures, or flail chest. These suggest the presence of an underlying pulmonary contusion. Crackles may be heard on auscultation but are rarely heard in the emergency room and are nonspecific. Patients with pulmonary contusions should be referred to a physician for further evaluation.

STERNAL FRACTURE/CONTUSION

Sternal fractures result from a high-impact blunt trauma to the chest. While it is more common in automobile accidents than in sports, it can still occur in sports. Sports emergency care personnel must be aware of this injury because it can result in an injury to the underlying cardiac muscle.

Clinical signs and symptoms of this injury may be point tenderness over the sternum that will worsen with deep inspiration or forceful expiration. Signs of shock may indicate an injury to the underlying tissue. In the field, it is difficult sometimes to differentiate between the sternal contusion and fracture, and an x-ray will help make the differential diagnosis.

RIB FRACTURES AND CONTUSIONS

Rib contusions are common in sports. These injuries occur more frequently in collision sports like football, hockey, lacrosse, and wrestling but can also occur is other sports. A direct blow to the rib cage can contuse intercostal muscles or fracture them if the blow is severe enough.

Because the intercostal muscles are essential to breathing, the patient/athlete may experience sharp pain with expiration, inspiration, coughing, laughing, or sneezing. There will be point tenderness over the rib cage and pain with compression of the rib cage.

Rib fractures are especially common in collision sports. Fractures can be caused by direct and indirect trauma. Ribs 5 through 9 are the most commonly fractured.

The direct-blow rib fracture causes the most serious damage because the external force fractures and displaces the ribs inward. Such a mechanism may completely displace the bone and cause fragmentation. The fragments may cut, tear, or perforate the tissue of the pleurae (hemothorax) or they may collapse one lung (pneumothorax). Contrary to the direct injury, the indirect fracture usually causes the rib to fracture outward, producing an oblique or transverse fracture. Stress fractures can also occur. Repetitive movements like throwing or rowing or repetitive coughing or sneezing can result in a rib stress fracture.

Rib fractures are either easily detectable due to a deformity or difficult to detect. An athlete should always be examined thoroughly for any underlying conditions that may occur. The athlete should be stabilized and immediately transported to a medical facility if there is a possibility of an unstable fracture.

COSTOCHONDRAL SEPARATION/DISLOCATION

Costochondral separations occur from a direct blow to the anterolateral aspect of the thorax or indirectly from a sudden twist or fall on a ball that compresses the rib cage.

The costochondral injury displays many signs that are similar to the rib fracture, with the exception of the location of the pain. The pain location of this injury will be localized in the junction of the rib cartilage and rib. The athlete will complain of sharp pain with sudden movement of the trunk and difficulty breathing deeply. There is point tenderness.

Management of costochondral separations and dislocations includes ice and referral to a physician for follow-up

THORACIC SPINE FRACTURE

Thoracic spinal fractures can occur whenever forces exceed the strength and stability of the spinal column. Thoracic spine fractures are uncommon in sports but need to be recognized because spinal cord injuries represent the second most serious long-term morbidities resulting from thoracic trauma, with traumatic aortic rupture being the first.

Fractures most commonly occur in the lower thoracic vertebrae and are less common in the upper and mid-thoracic vertebrae. The ribs and the orientation of the facets stabilize the upper thoracic spine (T1–T10). However, at the T12–L1 junction, increased range of motion allows combinations of acute hyperflexion and rotation. The mechanisms of thoracolumbar spine trauma are hyperflexion, vertical compression, hyperextension, and shearing injury.

Hyperflexion injury includes flexion with compression, lateral flexion, flexion-rotation, and flexion-distraction injuries. These mechanisms can occur in collision sports and some noncontact sports. A vertical compression mechanism results in burst injuries of the vertebral body. Hyperextension injuries result in posterior spinal compression fractures, while shearing injury can cause subluxation or dislocation of the spinal column.

The athlete may experience the following signs and symptoms with a thoracic spine injury: pain or point tenderness in the thoracic region or paralysis below the chest or waist. The lower extremities may be cool.

Management of Thoracic Spine Injury/Trauma

- Maintain spinal immobilization.
- Establish an open airway.
- Activate EMS.
- Treat for shock.
- Administer high concentration oxygen.
- Monitor oxygen saturation with a pulse oximeter.
- Transport the athlete rapidly to a hospital.
- Notify medical direction.

Conclusion

Most thoracic injuries, although rare in sports, can be life threatening in nature. It is important to recognize these life-threatening conditions because it is vital that the athlete receives prompt intervention, EMS activation, and transport to the nearest hospital. It is extremely important that most of the injuries in this chapter are recognized by the sports medicine team and treated properly in the field because it may help save the athlete's life.

Bibliography

Arnheim DD. *Principles of Athletic Training.* Boston, Mass: McGraw Hill; 2000.

Campbell JE. BTLS, *Basic Trauma Life Support for the EMT-B and The First Responder.* Upper Saddle River, NJ: Pearson Prentice Hall; 2004.

Ciocca M. Pneumothorax in a weight lifter. *Physician and Sportsmedicine.* 2000;28(4):97-103.

Curtin SM, Tucker AM, Gens DR. Pneumothorax in sports. *Physician and Sportsmedicine.* 2000;28(8):23-32.

Copass MK, Gonzales L, Eisenberg MS, Soper RG. *EMT Manual.* Philadelphia: WB Saunders Company; 1998.

Micheli LJ. *The Sports Medicine Bible.* New York: Harper Perennial; 1995.

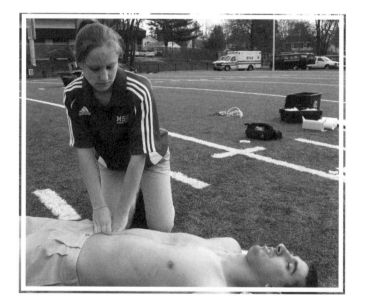

Chapter 10 Abdominal and Pelvic Injuries

David A. Middlemas, EdD, ATC

It is not unusual for individuals participating in physical activity to have emergencies involving the abdominal and pelvic regions. Athletes and others participating in exercise are subject to pain and discomfort resulting from injuries or illness involving the internal organs of the abdomen. The sports medicine team members providing emergency care for individuals participating in sports need to be aware of the potential causes of abdominal problems in athletes, their signs and symptoms, and the sports medicine team member's role in recognizing the nature and extent of injury so the athlete can be referred for appropriate medical care.

Many sports and physical activities involve intentional and unintentional collisions with other athletes, impact with sports implements, and high-velocity movement and twisting. The ability of the sports emergency care team member to recognize and interpret the effects of events in exercise and sports on the internal organs of the abdomen is essential to determining the extent of injury and the need for immediate action. This chapter will provide the reader with an overview of the anatomy of the abdominopelvic region, assessment of abdominal injuries, and medical conditions and guidelines for immediate care.

Review of Clinically Relevant Anatomy

The abdominal cavity is the area below the thoracic cavity that contains many of the body's internal organs. It is separated from the thorax by the diaphragm and lined with a membrane called peritoneum. The lower portion of the abdominal cavity surrounded by the pelvis, vertebra, and sacrum is called the pelvic region (Figure 10-1).

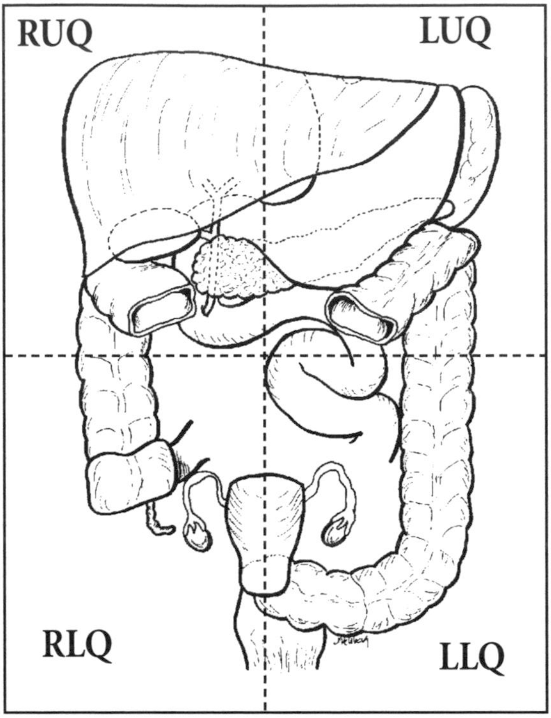

Figure 10-1. The abdominopelvic cavity. (Illustration by Joelle Rehberg, DO.)

The location of the organs in the abdomen and pelvis is usually described by dividing the abdomen into 4 quadrants. The abdominal quadrants are defined by drawing a vertical and horizontal line through the navel. The quadrants and the structures located within them are shown in Figure 10-1. The quadrants are called the left upper quadrant (LUQ), right upper quadrant (RUQ), left lower quadrant (LLQ), and right lower quadrant (RLQ). The quality of communication between medical professionals and the accuracy of injury records is improved when everyone involved in the care of the injured athlete uses the same terminology.

The liver, gall bladder, spleen, pancreas, and the digestive organs (stomach, small intestine, and large intestine) are contained in the abdominal cavity. The urinary bladder and female reproductive organs are in the pelvic region, with male genitalia being external. It is important to note that the kidneys are not within the abdomen. They are located outside the peritoneum behind the abdominal cavity, covered by the muscles of the back and protected by the lower ribs.

To assist in understanding the nature of emergencies in the abdominopelvic region and their implications, it is important to understand the basic structure

Table 10-1

CATEGORIES OF ORGANS OF THE ABDOMINAL AND PELVIC CAVITIES

Solid Organs	Hollow Organs	Reproduction
Liver	Stomach	Female: ovaries, uterus, and vagina
Spleen	Small intestine	Male: scrotum, testes, and penis
Pancreas	Large intestine	
Kidney	Gall bladder	
	Urinary bladder	

and functions of the organs in this region. It is helpful to divide the organs into the following categories: hollow organs and solid organs (Table 10-1).

Hollow organs either allow materials to pass through them, as in the stomach and intestines, or serve as "holding tanks" for materials until they are needed or expelled from the body, as in the gall bladder or urinary bladder. As a rule, hollow organs tend to be injured less in sports and physical activity because they are at significantly less risk when they are empty. The best way to prevent injuries to the hollow organs is to have them as empty as possible when participating in sports or exercise. Such things as not eating immediately before competition and urinating before a game or practice significantly reduce the risk of injury to digestive organs and the urinary bladder.

Solid organs do not have cavities inside them to hold or store fluids. They tend to have significant blood supplies that are necessary to complete their functions. The solid organs include the liver, spleen, pancreas, kidneys, ovaries, and testes. The very fact that these organs will not easily compress when suffering a collision, combined with their ample blood supply, place them at a higher risk of bruising or tearing with potentially life-threatening bleeding.

The liver, primarily located in the RUQ, is the largest solid organ of the body. It has many functions, including making bile, converting glucose to glycogen for storage, producing urea, and storing multiple substances for the body. As a result of these critical functions, it has a very rich blood supply. Injuries to the liver can result in serious bruising or significant bleeding into the abdominal cavity.

The spleen is located in the LUQ of the abdomen. Its job is to filter blood and to store red blood cells and platelets. It has a plentiful blood supply and is at risk for injury from blows to the upper abdomen. It is also important to note that the spleen swells in individuals who have had mononucleosis, thus increasing the risk of injury from contact or collision.

Although the kidneys are located outside the abdominal cavity, their function of producing urine is critical to the body. The kidneys, which are on the back of the body, are somewhat protected by the ribs. The process of filtering waste products from the blood produces urine. It then flows through the ureters to the urinary bladder, which is located in the lower abdominal cavity. Because the kidneys are the primary filters that remove waste from the bloodstream, they have a very rich blood supply. Although the lower ribs cover the kidneys, blows to the kidneys can cause significant injuries.

The majority of reproductive organs in women are within the abdominal cavity. The ovaries, uterus, fallopian tubes, and vagina are internal, placing them at significantly less risk for injury than the male's external reproductive anatomy. The male reproductive anatomy is more likely to be injured from a direct blow or collision due to the fact that it is external. The penis, which has a rich blood supply, and the testes, which are solid, have little protection.

Avoiding Injury

Preventing abdominal injuries in athletes requires the efforts of many individuals. The sports emergency care team member (ie, athletic trainer, physician, nurse), coach, official, parents, and even the athlete him- or herself can be essential to preventing or reducing the occurrence of abdominal trauma in sports. By working together, everyone can ensure that athletes have the proper equipment, learn and use correct sports technique, and that rules are appropriately taught and enforced.

Protective equipment for the abdominal region includes such items as baseball and softball chest protectors and extensions for shoulder pads in sports such as football and ice hockey. In order to get the best protection possible, the coach and sports emergency care team member should work together to ensure that protective equipment is in good repair, meets required standards, and fits the athlete properly. The athlete is a critical link in helping to keep his or her equipment safe. Reporting damaged or ill-fitting equipment allows for immediate repair or adjustment of any problems before an injury occurs.

Proper technique in those sports where contact and collision are part of the game is essential to reducing injury. Coaches and officials can work together to reduce the occurrence of injury by teaching proper methods of contact and collision and to appropriately penalize those who abuse the rules.

Finally, there are times where the best method for preventing a potentially devastating situation is to disqualify an individual from participation in certain activities where the potential for injury is unacceptable for that person. Examples of situations in which a physician might disqualify an athlete from participation in collision or contact sports may include absence of a paired organ, such as a kidney or eye, or a medical condition that could place the athlete in danger. It may be appropriate in these situations to substitute an activity with lower risk of injury for the involved athlete.

Evaluation and Recognition of Abdominal Injuries

Many of the emergencies encountered in the athletic venue can be assessed by directly visualizing and touching the injured tissue. However, evaluation of injuries and medical conditions in the abdominal region requires the practitioner to apply knowledge and skills that will allow him or her to recognize emergencies without the ability to directly access the effected organ or tissue. This section will help the caregiver to understand the use of vital signs to recognize illnesses and injuries requiring indirect methods of evaluation.

We begin our discussion with an explanation of the concept of "indirect methods of evaluation." Unlike such things as open wounds or bruising, injuries to internal organs and structures require the caregiver to evaluate the status of an effected body part by looking at "something else." Usually that "something else" is one or more of the vital signs. The caveat here is that a victim who has been participating in exercise or sports will likely have vital signs that are different from those of a resting patient immediately before the injury occurs. These differences, which may be interpreted as abnormal for the average person, are the norm or baseline for determining the extent of injury in someone who was physically active at the time he or she was hurt. It is important for the emergency caregiver to be familiar with these differences as he or she begins the assessment. A summary of the differences is presented in Chapter 3.

In athletic situations, injuries to the abdomen usually involve a collision with another athlete, running into an object such as a wall or fence, or being struck by an athletic implement like a bat or stick. These impacts often occur in the course of play, and the injured athlete may or may not appear to be injured immediately after the incident. The primary concern in these situations is that of internal bleeding from damaged internal organs, especially those with ample blood supply, like the liver, spleen, and kidneys. Injuries to these structures have the potential to be life threatening and may require surgery. It is important for the sports emergency care team member to collect information quickly and efficiently in situations in which abdominal trauma may be present. Decisions relating to the possible extent of injury and immediate course of care will depend on the caregiver's ability to assess the situation and get the athlete to appropriate medical care in a timely fashion.

In the ideal situation, abdominal injury assessment begins with observation of the events leading up to the injury and the mechanism of injury. For example, a running back in football who is struck in the middle of the back with another player's helmet may have a kidney injury, or a lacrosse player who gets the butt of another player's stick thrust into the LUQ of the abdomen might have ruptured the spleen. In order to gain the most information from observing the events leading up to an injury, the caregiver must have an understanding of the anatomy of the injured body region and the possible injuries that can result from the event causing the injury.

It is not unusual for the sports emergency care team member to be called to the location of an injury after it has occurred. The disadvantage in these situations is that he or she was not able to witness the mechanism of injury. Information about how the injury occurred must be gathered by observing the injured athlete and surroundings as one approaches and by asking questions of the athlete, coaches, officials, and other players to determine how the accident happened and the extent of possible injuries. It is usually best to take the history using a structured interview format such as the SAMPLE history.

Like any emergency situation, the first concern of the caregiver is to assess the injured athlete for the presence of severe or potentially devastating injuries or conditions. When life-threatening problems such as absence of breathing or pulse or severe bleeding are present, the sports emergency care team member should take the appropriate actions to immediately deal with the problem. When the injured athlete is determined to be in no immediate danger, a more thorough examination, or secondary survey, that can focus on the potential abdominal injury should take place.

Understanding what caused the injury is particularly helpful when dealing with internal injuries because the sports emergency care team member must make decisions about injured organs that can not be directly seen or touched. The care provider should ask the patient where and how the blow to the abdomen took place and what the patient felt immediately at the time of injury. Questions about the nature and intensity of any pain, lightheadedness or dizziness, nausea, and any other abnormal feelings or sensations at the time of injury and afterward will help the rescuer get an overall understanding of the possibility of internal injury to the athlete.

After determining the mechanism of injury, one of the first concerns in assessing abdominal injuries is the location and nature of the patient's pain. Generally, the injured athlete will have pain at the location of the injury. For example, if a hockey player has an injury to the liver after being checked into the boards, one would expect pain in the RUQ of the abdomen; if the spleen is ruptured after being hit in the abdomen with a lacrosse stick, one would expect pain in the LUQ of the abdomen and so on. Victims of internal organ injuries may have pain or soreness at places away from the injured structure in addition to pain at the location of the injury. This phenomenon is called referred pain. Referred pain is a condition in which pain from an injury or illness in one part of the body presents in another location of the body. One example is Kehr's sign, which is a referred pain pattern for an injury to the spleen in which the patient will have pain or soreness in the left shoulder. Some referred pain patterns are presented in Figure 10 2.

Questions about lightheadedness, nausea, and changes in sensations around the abdomen provide information about whether or not there might be internal bleeding from injured structures in the abdomen. Because any bleeding from abdominal injuries cannot be directly observed, the caregiver must look for signs and symptoms that indicate the presence of secondary conditions caused by the internal bleeding. A secondary condition is one that occurs as a result of an injury or illness existing in the body. The most significant secondary condition when it comes to suspecting the possibility of internal bleeding is shock, of which lightheadedness, dizziness, and nausea are symptoms.

Remember that a comprehensive patient history will collect information from the athlete, the other players in the area, officials, and coaches about the causes of the injury and the patient's condition. The answers to questions about what happened, the presence and nature of any pain, and other feelings or sensations help the caregiver understand the potential severity of the injury and set the basis for the hands-on portion of the patient assessment.

The Physical Examination

The sports emergency care team member will conduct a physical assessment after collecting information about the nature and cause of the injury to verify what was learned in the history and to pinpoint the specific structures that may have been injured. The physical examination should assess appropriate vital signs and include palpation of the abdomen.

A primary concern of the sports emergency care team member when caring for patients with potential internal bleeding from injuries to solid internal organs, like the liver and spleen, is the onset of shock. The sports emergency care team member should be prepared to assess the rate and quality of the athlete's pulse and respirations. It is also important to assess the victim's blood pressure. As with any other bleeding injury, changes in vital signs provide information about the patient's current status and the stability of his or her condition. Vital sign assessment should focus on changes that indicate the possibility of internal bleeding such as a weak rapid pulse, changes in rate and quality of breathing, drop in blood pressure, pale skin, and sweating. Patients with significant blood loss may also present with changes in their level of consciousness consistent with those of patients in shock.

Injuries to hollow organs present the additional problem of leakage of their contents into the abdominal cavity. The presence of such things as urine or bowel contents in the abdominal cavity creates the additional dangers of significant infection in the abdominal region and inflammation and irritation of the lining of the cavity. This is called peritonitis. The sports emergency care team member may find elevated body temperature, elevated skin

Figure 10-2. Referred pain patterns. (Reprinted with permission from O'Connor DP. *Clinical Pathology for Athletic Trainers: Recognizing Systemic Disease.* Thorofare, NJ: SLACK Incorporated; 2001:82–83.)

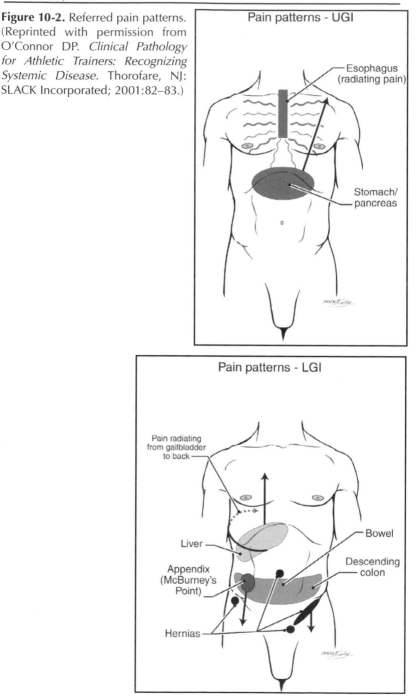

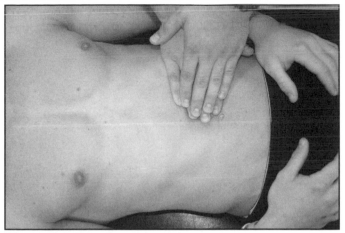

Figure 10-3. Palpation of the abdomen.

temperature, and severe abdominal pain. These conditions may require surgery and/or the administration of antibiotics by the physician, and—if not treated promptly—may be life threatening.

Palpation of the abdomen (Figure 10-3) can be very helpful in determining the nature and extent of injuries to the region. Abdominal assessment should include the ability to recognize guarding, abdominal rigidity, and rebound tenderness. Guarding occurs when the athlete tightens the muscles of the abdominal wall when the sport emergency care team member applies pressure to the abdomen at a point where the athlete has pain. Guarding can be an indication of acute abdominal pain and/or inflammation to internal organs. Guarding serves as an attempt to protect the area from additional aggravation. Abdominal rigidity presents as contraction of the muscular walls of the abdomen so that the abdomen feels firm or hard to the touch of the evaluator. It can indicate swelling in the abdomen, possibly related to bleeding, abdominal pain, or patient apprehension about being touched. Pain upon quickly releasing the abdominal wall after slow pressure is called rebound tenderness. It is an indicator of pain in the abdominal lining and happens in response to the rapid stretching of the irritated tissue after pressure. It is a sign commonly found in individuals with acute appendicitis.

Abdominal and Pelvic Injuries

Direct blows to the abdomen can result in injuries ranging from surface contusions and muscle bruises to significant internal organ damage. This section will present some of the common abdominal injuries, their common causes, and how they usually present.

Blows to the anterior surface of the abdomen tend to cause injuries to the organs and structures in the abdominal cavity where the impact took place. Because solid organs such as the liver and spleen are located in the upper 2 quadrants of the abdomen, internal bleeding is of particular concern when the athlete is struck at that location. Staying with the classification of internal injuries into those involving either solid or hollow organs, let us first look at how injuries to some of the solid organs might present themselves.

SOLID ORGAN INJURIES

The spleen is located under the stomach in the LUQ of the abdomen. Contusions or rupture of the spleen can occur as a result of a direct blow to the LUQ. Athletic activities that might result in injury to the spleen include such things as tackling in football, collisions or checking in ice hockey, or being struck in the abdomen with a sports implement such as a stick or bat. The victim will have pain in the LUQ. In addition, spleen injuries can also have Kehr's sign. If the spleen is ruptured, there will be internal bleeding, which may be delayed by the organ's ability to splint itself. When this happens, internal bleeding, and hence the signs and symptoms of shock, begin some time after the injury takes place. Patient evaluation will often reveal tenderness in the LUQ, possibly rebound tenderness, nausea, and signs and symptoms of shock. Athletes in contact and collision sports with medical conditions such as mononucleosis are at increased risk of spleen injury due to enlargement of the organ. Physician clearance should be obtained before these athletes return to their sports activities.

The liver is the largest solid organ in the body. It occupies the majority of the RUQ and is susceptible to contusion or laceration from direct blows to the abdomen. Like the spleen, it is highly vascularized and injuries have the potential to bleed into the abdomen relatively quickly. Victims of a lacerated liver may have pain on deep palpation, rebound tenderness, and nausea and can develop signs and symptoms of shock fairly quickly. Referred pain may present in the center of the chest and under the left arm.

Blows to the back can cause injury to the kidneys. Contusions or lacerations to the kidneys can result in internal bleeding. Often an injury to the kidney will present with localized pain over the "flank" that may be intense and burning. Palpation of the back in the area of the kidneys can elicit tenderness. The victim of a kidney contusion or laceration might also have a burning sensation while urinating, blood in his or her urine (hematuria), loss of the ability to urinate, and/or referred pain in the lower abdominal region.

HOLLOW ORGAN INJURIES

Injuries to hollow organs like the urinary bladder, stomach, and intestines can usually be prevented by having them as empty as possible before activities with the potential for collisions or contact. Although some bleeding can occur with injuries to these organs, the main concern is the spilling of contents into the abdominal cavity, causing inflammation, infection, and peritonitis. Generally speaking, these victims will present with abdominal pain; tenderness on palpation; abdominal guarding; and signs and symptoms of inflammation and infection, including fever and soreness. There may also be nausea and vomiting.

An injury to the urinary bladder can occur from a direct blow to the midline in the pelvic region. Spilling of urine into the abdominal cavity can cause severe pain and inflammation in the lower abdomen.

Open wounds in the abdominal cavity or those involving penetrating objects present the possibility of internal bleeding and infection. Open abdominal injuries can occur from sports implements such as the javelin or a ski pole or collisions with equipment such as metal fence posts.

Injuries to the genitalia can occur in sports in which there is the possibility of being struck in the groin area by a ball or sports implement or in a collision with another athlete. Because the majority of female reproductive organs are internal, genital injuries in female athletes are not very common in sports. Direct blows to the genital area can cause contusions or lacerations, which the sports emergency care team member can care for using ice or appropriate bandaging. The sports emergency care team member should take care to protect the privacy or modesty of the victim at all times by moving to a private area or covering the athlete with a blanket or other available item. Males, on the other hand, have a higher risk of genital injury because the anatomy is outside the abdominal cavity. Injuries to male genitalia include contusions to the scrotum, testes, and penis; testicular torsion; and laceration or entrapment of anatomy in clothing or equipment. Athletes participating in activities in which there is a risk of injury to the external genitalia should be required to wear a cup protector.

Blows to the groin area can result in painful injuries to the external anatomy in males. It is not uncommon for contusions and lacerations to happen as a result of being hit by another athlete, a ball, or sports implement. Lacerations to the penis are of concern because of the rich blood supply in the area and thus they have the potential to bleed freely. Lacerations to the scrotum can be superficial or deep enough to expose and damage the testicle. Superficial wounds that are bleeding can be treated the same as any other laceration, taking care to preserve the victim's dignity. Deeper lacerations involving the penis or scrotum should be considered emergent and the athlete transported by ambulance to the emergency room.

Closed injuries to the male genitals can be very serious. A direct blow to the groin can result in deep contusion or fracture of a testicle or tearing of a blood vessel in the scrotum. In either case the situation is an emergency. Disruption of blood supply to the testicle can possibly result in loss of the organ if not cared for by a physician immediately and properly. These sorts of injuries present with significant pain in the scrotal area accompanied by significant swelling in the scrotum and require immediate transportation to the emergency room.

Testicular torsion is a medical emergency that can result in loss of blood supply and possibly result in loss of the testicle. In this condition the testicle can rotate in the scrotum. When this happens, the blood supply can be cut off. The patient complains of sudden pain and swelling on one side of the scrotum or in one of the testes. Testicular torsion is often the result of a predisposing situation in which the testicle is not adequately attached to the inside of the scrotum. This condition is seen most frequently in boys but has been seen in adults. The condition must be addressed promptly with surgery to restore the blood supply.

Emergency Care of Abdominal and Pelvic Injuries

When suspecting abdominal injury, it is important to continue monitoring the patient's vital signs for changes that would indicate the possibility of internal bleeding. The sports emergency care team member should evaluate the injured athlete's pulse, respirations, skin color and temperature, and—when possible—blood pressure. Weak, rapid pulse; rapid, shallow breathing; pale, cool, and clammy skin; and decreased blood pressure are all indicators of internal bleeding that will send the patient into shock. The injured athlete may also complain of nausea and dizziness and may vomit.

Once an abdominal injury is suspected, the following steps should be taken:

- Activate EMS.
- Place the victim in a comfortable position. The recovery position will assist in maintaining a patent airway in the event the patient is nauseated or vomits.
- Treat for shock. If the victim does not have a spinal or head injury, elevate the feet and legs. Maintain the athlete's body temperature by using a blanket, jacket, or some other covering when necessary.

It is important that the victim's vital signs be assessed for changes at regular intervals while waiting for the ambulance and during transportation to the hospital. Do not give the injured athlete anything to eat or drink because internal injuries may require surgery. Because the sports emergency care team member is not able to control internal bleeding directly, it is important to be prepared to provide basic life support in the event the patient's condition should worsen significantly.

There are times when an athlete may suffer an abdominal injury with an impaled object. One example of this would be an individual struck in the abdomen with a javelin. As with all injuries involving impaled objects, it is important to leave the object in place, pad it, and bandage it where it is. The caregiver must continue to be aware that the visible injury is complicated by the possibility that the javelin (or other object) is also penetrating an internal organ and that moving it could result in significant internal bleeding.

An additional consideration with an impaled sports implement like a javelin is that it may not fit into the back of the ambulance. In rare cases, the sports emergency care team may need to summon rescue personnel for assistance in cutting the impaled object to a length that will allow the victim to be safely transported with it bandaged in place. Professional rescue personnel will have access to specialized equipment such as the "Jaws of Life," which can cut the post or implement with as little movement as possible.

Common Medical Emergencies in the Abdomen and Pelvis

There will be times when athletes will have abdominal pain or discomfort that is not a result of an injury or collision. Although the sports emergency care team member can not directly treat the cause of the problem, assessment and recognition of medical conditions in the abdomen can prevent significant problems. Timely awareness of potentially serious illness will allow the athlete to be referred to a physician for rapid diagnosis and treatment.

The patient is said to have an acute abdomen when he or she suddenly develops abdominal pain. Conditions that can lead to abdominal pain or discomfort can be relatively minor or they can be severe. A physician will be able to determine if the pain can be alleviated through medication and conservative treatment or whether the patient requires more invasive care, such as surgery.

EVALUATING AND RECOGNIZING MEDICAL CONDITIONS IN THE ABDOMEN

The sports emergency care team member should observe the patient for signs indicating the location and intensity of pain. Facial expression, sweating, and posture provide information about the severity of the pain. The athlete may be lying on his or her side with knees drawn up to try to alleviate the pain. It is also important to take a history focusing on the abdomen in order to identify the possible causes of the pain.

The primary focus in taking a history for a person complaining of abdominal pain is the location, nature, and intensity of the pain (Table 10-2). The sports emergency care team member can easily remember what to ask the

Table 10-2

SUGGESTED OUTLINE FOR STRUCTURED INTERVIEW FOR ABDOMINAL INJURIES OR CONDITIONS

Abdominal Injury	Illness
What happened? (Were you hit? Was there a collision?)	Describe the problem.
Where were you hit?	Have you eaten anything you do not usually eat?
What did you feel at the time of injury?	Please list the symptoms.
Have you had this problem before? Are you nauseous? Have you vomited? Does it hurt?	

O	Onset	When did the problem begin? What caused it?
P	Provokes/Palliates	What makes it better? What makes it worse?
Q	Quality	Describe your pain (ie, is the pain sharp, dull, achy, burning?)
R	Region/Radiates	Where does it hurt? Does the pain move or spread?
S	Severity	Rate your pain on a scale from I to I0
T	Timing of the pain	Has it been constant? Does it come and go? How long has the pain been there?

patient by using OPQRST described in Chapter 3. This mnemonic serves as a reminder to ask about the Onset (the start of the problem), Provocation and Palliation (what makes it feel better or worse), Quality (sharp, dull, ache, burning), Region (where it hurts), Severity (how much it hurts), and the Timing of the pain. Information about nausea and vomiting, diarrhea, constipation, and fever often provides additional information that identifies the cause of the problem.

The patient's answers from the history will guide the sports emergency care team member in performing a physical exam concentrating on the abdomen. Take the patient's vital signs. The steps in the assessment process should be explained to the patient to reduce stress and apprehension. The 4 quadrants

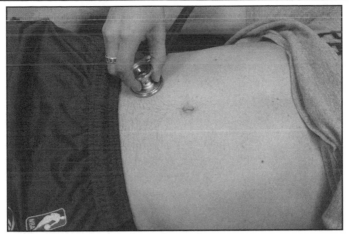

Figure 10-4. Assessing bowel sounds.

of the abdomen should be palpated. Begin away from the suspected location of the pain and work toward it. Gently press on the regions of the abdomen, feeling for rigidity and/or guarding. Ask the patient if he or she can relax the abdomen. When the location of the pain is identified, check for rebound tenderness. Note the results of the assessment and record the information so it can be communicated to the physician.

The sports emergency care team member can also quickly check to see if the patient's bowel sounds are present (Figure 10-4). The absence of normal bowel sounds can indicate the possibility of such problems as bowel obstruction or significant abdominal injury or illness. Place the head of the stethoscope on the anterior abdomen. Listen to all 4 quadrants of the abdomen. Normal bowel sounds include a combination of squeaking and gurgling sounds, indicating that intestinal contents are being moved through the digestive system. If the sounds are diminished or absent, the information should be recorded in the patient notes and communicated to the physician.

REDUCING THE LIKELIHOOD OF ABDOMINAL PAIN

Many of the nontraumatic causes of abdominal pain such as acute appendicitis, gall or kidney stones, and kidney or bladder infections result from medical conditions or emergencies that cannot be predicted by the patient. There are no effective prevention strategies that target these sorts of conditions. Basic common sense lifestyle choices such as a well-balanced diet, adequate hydration, and close attention to bodily changes can help reduce the chances of medically related problems.

Emergency Care
of the Acute Abdomen

The need for emergency transportation and treatment for an individual with abdominal pain would be dictated by the onset and severity of the pain, the possible underlying cause, and the stability of the patient's vital signs. Individuals with moderate to severe abdominal pain accompanied by vital sign changes such as altered pulse or blood pressure, fever, chills, nausea, vomiting, and/or signs of shock should be made as comfortable as possible and monitored while EMS is called. The location and nature of the pain may provide the sports emergency care team member with clues as to its possible cause, but definitive diagnosis and treatment by a physician are essential for these patients. Under these circumstances, the patient should be given nothing to eat or drink while waiting for the ambulance because it may aggravate the condition or make it more difficult in the event surgery is required.

In many cases, teenagers and adults with relatively minor episodes of abdominal pain or discomfort may have had it before. Such conditions as indigestion, irritable bowel syndrome, or menstrual cramps may be significant enough to affect an athlete's ability to exercise or compete, but they do not usually require emergency transportation and treatment. Athletes who do not have a history of abdominal discomfort should stop their activity, be made comfortable, and be referred to their physician for diagnosis and appropriate treatment. Those who have recurrent or chronic episodes of minor abdominal conditions may have already been advised by their health care provider on how to care for discomfort or minor pain when it occurs. In these situations it is appropriate to assist the athlete in following the instructions he or she has been given by the doctor.

The most effective method of determining the patient's knowledge regarding the abdominal discomfort or pain is by taking a comprehensive history related to the abdominal discomfort. Asking the athlete about when the pain started, the severity of the pain, and factors that worsen or lessen the pain can verify whether or not the episode is a recurrence of an existing problem or something new. Listening carefully to the patient's answers to questions can help the sports emergency care team member to identify whether or not the athlete is familiar with the problem. In any situation in which the athlete has had to stop participation due to abdominal pain or discomfort, it is appropriate to make sure a qualified medical professional has assessed him or her before returning to play. In situations in which the athlete is a minor, it is imperative that the parent or guardian be advised of the situation. In many cases, reviewing the options for follow-up with a physician provide the parent and athlete with information they need and a degree of comfort.

Other Medical Conditions of the Abdomen and Pelvis

The information in this section presents the signs and symptoms for common medical conditions of the abdomen. This information can help the sports emergency care team member in deciding the potential severity of the problem and the type of assistance that is needed.

Some causes of abdominal discomfort or pain are relatively minor and may resolve with little medical treatment. Other illnesses or conditions causing abdominal pain can be significant and may be life threatening if not diagnosed by a physician and treated properly. The role of the sports emergency care team member is to recognize signs and symptoms in the athlete that indicate potential abdominal illness and facilitate getting the patient to the appropriate medical professional in a timely fashion. Signs and symptoms of medical conditions in the abdomen are presented to provide background information for the sports emergency care team that helps them recognize the athlete's need for medical care.

Problems with the organs of the digestive system often give the patient abdominal pain. The pain can be burning, sharp, dull, or intense.

Dyspepsia is a term that describes pain in the upper abdomen that may come and go but is usually present the majority of the time. Common causes of dyspepsia are gastroesophageal reflux disease (GERD) and stomach ulcers. GERD is a condition in which acid from the stomach splashes out of the upper valve onto the walls of the esophagus. The patient will complain of burning pain in the mid-upper abdomen and/or heartburn. The pain may be constant but is sometimes relieved when the patient eats or takes an antacid. Occasional heartburn may not be a significant problem, but recurrent burning pain in the upper abdomen may be a sign of GERD, which has the potential to cause long-term damage to the esophagus. Stomach ulcers are wounds in the lining of the stomach. They may be caused by stress, a virus, or dietary concerns. Ulcers also present with abdominal pain, burping, nausea, and/or heartburn. The potential for significant bleeding exists if ulcers go untreated because they are open wounds in the stomach lining. A physician should evaluate persistent upper abdominal pain and burning in order to provide proper treatment.

Generalized abdominal pain can result from a number of conditions in the intestinal tract. Intestinal gas can cause significant pain in the abdomen that might be strong enough to cause an athlete to double over. Often "gas pains" are accompanied with increased bowel sounds, or "gurgling," and will resolve themselves.

Irritable bowel syndrome (IBS) is a term used to describe conditions that cause abdominal pain, diarrhea, and significant discomfort in the abdominal region. The term includes conditions like Crohn's disease and ulcerative colitis.

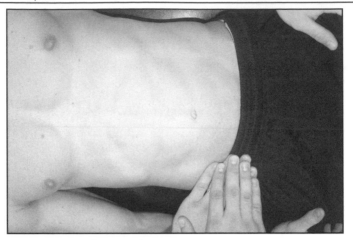

Figure 10-5. Palpation of McBurney's point.

Abdominal pain can also be caused by pockets or folds in the walls of the intestines, called diverticula, that become infected or inflamed, causing pain, nausea, vomiting, fever, and changes in bowel habits. A physician should properly diagnose and treat an athlete with frequent instances of abdominal pain that persist for a prolonged period of time.

Infection and inflammation of the appendix can cause significant abdominal pain, nausea, vomiting, diarrhea, and fever. Acute appendicitis is often identified by pain in the RLQ of the abdomen, referred pain to the area of the navel, and rebound tenderness at the location of the appendix, called McBurney's point (Figure 10-5). Failure to recognize the signs and symptoms of appendicitis can allow the problem to progress as the infected appendix continues to swell and fill with pus. If left untreated, the appendix will eventually rupture, spreading the infections contents into the abdomen. When this happens, the patient has a potentially life-threatening condition that causes inflammation to the peritoneal lining and serious infection to the abdominal cavity.

There are medical conditions that do not present as emergencies, but the members of the sports emergency care team may be the first to whom the athlete reports the onset of symptoms relating to the illness. Listening to the pattern of symptoms and performing an initial assessment to determine the potential severity of the condition can be essential to preventing the progression of a condition to a serious problem.

An athlete with discomfort or pain in the RUQ with referred pain to the right shoulder may be suffering from an inflamed gall bladder (cholecystitis) or gall stones. The pain can be aggravated by fatty foods as bile is essential to their digestion. The individual may also have nausea and vomiting, depending on the severity of the condition.

An individual with unexplained abdominal pain, joint ache, fever, loss of appetite, nausea or vomiting, and fatigue may have contracted hepatitis. Hepatitis is a disease that affects the liver and is most often caused by a virus. There are 5 types of hepatitis. Hepatitis type A is the most common in the United States, but cases of type B and C are not uncommon. Hepatitis is contagious and is spread through such routes as unsanitary conditions, blood, feces, and sexual contact. The cause of the symptoms and the proper course of care must be determined by the physician after proper diagnostic testing.

Medical conditions of the urinary tract involve the kidneys, ureters, and bladder. Infections in the urinary tract can present with pain in the lower abdominal region and pubic area. Athletes with kidney infections can have low back soreness or pain, fever, and difficulty urinating. Infections in the urinary bladder, ureters, and/or urethra can cause pain or burning during urination.

The development of kidney stones can cause pain in the flank region of the back that radiates to the genital area. The pain can become severe and even disabling. Abnormal urinary habits and painful urination often occur in patients with kidney stones. Physician intervention is necessary to resolve the problem using one or more of many available treatment methods.

Abdominal pain may present in the female athlete as part of her normal menstrual cycle. Pain in the lower middle portion of the abdominopelvic region may occur in the middle of the menstrual cycle, which is associated with release of the egg from the ovary, or may occur with cramping during the menstrual period. The severity of the pain and cramping varies with the individual. When assessing a female athlete with lower abdominal pain, she is usually able to provide information relating to her normal pattern of pain and cramping during the menstrual cycle.

Sometimes abdominal pain in girls or women is due to medical conditions requiring the attention of their general physician or gynecologist. Patients who develop ovarian cysts can have severe pain in the abdominal or pelvic region and may also present with vaginal bleeding, nausea, and fever. Athletes who suddenly develop these symptoms should be treated as a medical emergency.

Ectopic pregnancy occurs when the fertilized egg implants in the wall of the fallopian tube outside the uterus. Women with a possible ectopic pregnancy can become dizzy and faint, develop low blood pressure, and have vaginal bleeding. It is important to tactfully ask female patients whether they may be pregnant during the history portion of the examination to rule out the possibility of gynecological causes for abdominal pain or symptoms.

We would be remiss in not providing a short discussion of the possibility of sexually transmitted diseases (STD) in the athletic population. The likelihood that sexually active individuals will be seeking the advice and treatment from sports medicine professionals they trust supports the need to recognize the signs of a potential STD. When the athlete communicates the onset of lesions, sores, or unusual skin problems on the genitals; unusual discharges from the penis or vagina; or pain during urination or intercourse, he or she may be communicating the presence of symptoms of STD. The sports emergency care team member should maintain the confidence and dignity of the athlete while strongly encouraging or requiring him or her to seek appropriate medical care for the condition. Since STDs are contagious, strongly encouraging medical follow-up and care provides appropriate care for the athlete and anyone with whom he or she has intimate contact.

Conclusion

The role of the sports emergency care team member or other emergency responder in dealing with emergencies in the abdomen and pelvic regions is to identify the potential causes of the athlete's problem and select the appropriate course of immediate care and referral for medical treatment. In order to be able to provide the best on-site care for the athlete, one should possess the ability to assess victims of both abdominal trauma and those whose abdominal pain may be due to medical conditions. The sports emergency care team member's ability to recognize the signs of significant abdominal injury or illness provides the basis for sound decision making and access to prompt emergency care.

The potential effects of internal bleeding or infection due to such conditions such as a ruptured appendix can be minimized by rapid identification of the problem's cause through effective assessment and immediate access to medical care. Daily contact between the athlete and the sports emergency care team member or other emergency care provider can play the most important role in early recognition of significant abdominal injury or illness by providing the athlete with a trusted professional to whom he or she can go immediately when discomfort, pain, or injury occur.

Bibliography

Abdominal Trauma, Evaluation of Penetrating Abdominal Trauma. Trauma.org Abdominal Trauma website. 2004. Available at: http://www.trauma.org/abdo/penetrating.html. Accessed October 24, 2006.

American Red Cross. *Emergency Response.* Yardley, Pa: Staywell Publishing; 2001.

American Urological Association. Testicular torsion. 2002. Available at: http://www.urologyhealth.org/search/index.cfm?search=testicular%20AND%20Torsion&searchtype=and&topic=134. Accessed October 21, 2006.

Booher JM, Thibodeau GA. *Athletic Injury Assessment.* 4th ed. New York: McGraw Hill; 2000.

Cuppett M, Walsh K. *General Medical Conditions in the Athlete.* St. Louis, Mo: Mosby; 2005.

Finch R, Banting SW. Commentary: modern management of splenic injury. *ANZ Journal of Surgery*. 2004;74(7):513.

Klepac SR, Samett EJ. Spleen. Available at: http://www.emedicine.com/radio/ topic645.htm. Accessed November 1, 2006

Kluger Y, Paul DB, Raves JJ, et al. Delayed rupture of the spleen—myths, facts, and their importance: case reports and literature review. *J Trauma*. 1994;36(4):568-571.

Limmer D, O'Keefe M, Dickinson EV, Grant H, Murray B, Bergeron JD. *Emergency Care*. 10 ed. New York: Prentice Hall; 2005.

Pollak AN, ed. *Emergency Care and Transportation of the Sick and Injured*. 9th ed. Boston, Mass: Jones and Bartlett Publishers; 2005.

Prentice WE. *Arnheim's Principles of Athletic Training*. 12th ed. New York: McGraw Hill; 2006.

Tamparo CD, Lewis MA. *Diseases of the Human Body*. 3rd ed. Philadelphia: FA Davis; 2000.

Wright JA. Seven abdominal assessment signs every emergency nurse should know. *Journal of Emergency Nursing*. 1997;23(5):446-450.

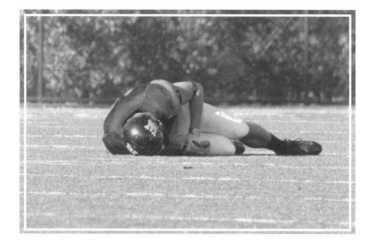

Chapter 11

Fractures and Soft Tissue Injuries

Michael Prybicien, MA, ATC, EMT-B, CSCS and Louis Rizio III, MD

Fractures, dislocations, and soft tissue injuries are among the most common injuries sustained in sports. This chapter aims to provide a straightforward approach to understanding injuries to bone and soft tissue, and the initial evaluation and management of such injuries. Proper initial evaluation and management are critical to ensure the athlete receives the proper medical attention, gets transferred to the hospital for further evaluation when appropriate, and most importantly is protected from further harm.

Review of Clinically Relevant Anatomy

BONE

This chapter will focus on bones of the extremities. Information on spinal anatomy can be found in Chapter 6. The bones of the arms and legs are long bones, each composed of an epiphyseal, metaphyseal, and diaphyseal segment (Figure 11-1). The epiphyseal segment is the portion of the bone that forms one side of a joint and is typically covered with articular cartilage. The metaphyseal segment is adjacent to the epiphyseal segment. The epiphyseal and metaphyseal segments fuse together once the individual reaches skeletal maturity. In childhood, bone growth occurs at the growth plate, which is between the epiphyseal, metaphyseal, and diaphyseal segments. The diaphyseal segment is the shaft of the long bone and is very strong.

Diaphyseal bone is composed of cortical bone, which is very strong and supports the body's weight. Metaphyseal bone tends to be wider and less tubular in appearance and is the portion of the long bone that forms one end

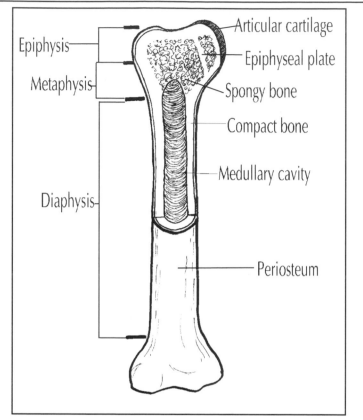

Epiphysis

Metaphysis

Diaphysis

Articular cartilage

Epiphyseal plate

Spongy bone

Compact bone

Medullary cavity

Periosteum

Figure 11-1. Bone. (Illustration by Joelle Rehberg, DO.)

of a joint. This metaphyseal bone is composed of cancellous bone and is not as strong as cortical bone.

JOINTS

The joints of the extremities are called synovial joints. The joint is formed by the proximal end of one bone and the distal end of another bone and is held together by a capsule and ligaments. The ends of each bone are covered with articular cartilage, which provides a low friction surface for motion and also a cushion for shock absorption. The connection of the 2 bones in this type of arrangement allows for motion of the joint; the ligaments and capsule provide stability (Figure 11-2). The capsule of the joint can be divided into a fibrous (outer) layer and synovial membrane (inner) layer. The ligaments that hold the joint stable are often thickenings of the fibrous layer made of dense collagen.

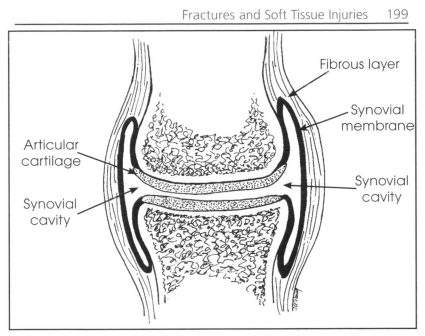

Figure 11-2. Synovial joint. (Illustration by Joelle Rehberg, DO.)

The synovial layer makes synovial fluid that bathes and nourishes the cartilage surfaces of the bones forming the joint.

SOFT TISSUE

Soft tissue is a broad term that can be used to describe many tissues in the musculoskeletal system. While the skin can be considered soft tissue and will be covered in the wound management section of this chapter, for the purposes of this section soft tissue refers to ligaments, tendons, and muscle. All of these structures are composed predominantly of collagen, but the type of collagen varies between the tissues. These soft tissues are critical for the normal functioning and action of joints. These structures allow for motion and stability of the joints they cross.

Ligaments usually attach on either side of the joint and connect one bone to another. Their major function is to provide stability to the joint it crosses. Injury to a ligament is termed a "sprain." It is a good idea to keep terminology accurate, especially when communicating with other members of the health care system; this avoids confusion and will hopefully convey the message most effectively.

Tendons are the connection between bone and muscle. It is the tendon attachment to bone that allows a muscle to move a joint. Muscle tissue

Figure 11-3. Immobilization of wrist and forearm injuries using a SAM splint.

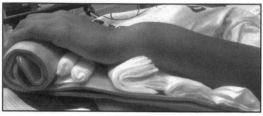

shortens (contracts) under voluntary control to produce movement. Injury to the tendon or muscle is termed a "strain." Tearing of a tendon can lead to inability to move an extremity or joint, especially if completely torn.

Fractures

"Is it broken or just fractured?" There is no distinction between breaks and fractures; they are one in the same. The disruption of the bone's continuity is what defines this injury. Fracture can occur from a direct blow or a rotational (twisting) injury without contact.

EVALUATION

The typical signs of a fracture are pain, swelling, and tenderness over the area. Movement of the extremity will aggravate the athlete's symptoms, and he or she cannot often bear weight on the lower extremity or move the upper extremity due to discomfort. Loss of function of the extremity is usually apparent.

Initial assessment of an injured and potentially fractured extremity includes a careful inspection of the limb, especially the skin. The clothing should be removed around the injured limb for complete inspection. Any wounds over the painful area should be considered indicative of an open (compound) fracture. Deformity may be present, indicating severe malalignment or displacement of the fractured ends (Figure 11-3). Tenderness over the bone is usually present and sometimes motion can be felt between the fractured ends; this is highly suspicious of a fracture.

A careful assessment of vascular supply and nerve function distal to the injury is vital. Sensory function is assessed grossly by determining the athlete's ability to feel the examiner's touch. This should be done on all surfaces of the limb circumferentially. In addition, an assessment of muscle function below the injury level is performed to determine motor nerve function. For example, ability to move all the toes or fingers up and down can give a gross estimate of nerve function. Any loss of sensation or movement below the injury needs to be documented prior to any splinting or immobilization.

Table 11-1

EMERGENCY MANAGEMENT
OF AN OPEN FRACTURE

* Cover the wound with Betadine (Purdue Products LP, Stamford, Conn) (iodine)- or alcohol-soaked gauze bandage.
* Immobilize the limb.
* Transfer the patient to the hospital immediately. (Infection risk increases if not treated within the first 6 hours!)

Vascular status or circulation is evaluated as well. Pulses should be felt below the level of the injury. In addition, a cold, very white (pallor), or blue extremity signals severe injury to the blood supply of the extremity. Capillary refill is not a reliable method of determining adequacy of the blood supply to the limb. All pulses felt or not felt need to be documented prior to transfer or immobilization.

INITIAL TREATMENT

If a fracture is suspected of the lower extremity, carrying the athlete off the field or assisting with ambulation to prevent weightbearing on the injured extremity is necessary. A splint or immobilization device is utilized to protect the injured extremity from undue motion. Typically, it is best to immobilize on the field as far above and below the area in question as possible. A good rule of thumb is to immobilize a joint above and below the injured area. The athlete should be sent for confirmatory X-rays. Examples of basic extremity splinting will be presented at the end of the chapter.

FRACTURE EMERGENCIES

An open (compound) fracture is an orthopaedic emergency and the athlete should be sent to the hospital for immediate treatment, which includes thorough operative irrigation and removal (debridement) of dirt, debris, or foreign material (ie, clothing pieces); stabilization; and antibiotics by intravenous administration. Initial management of an open fracture is listed in Table 11-1.

Loss of circulation to a limb is uncommon, but it needs to be corrected as soon as possible. When severe deformity exists to a limb and the circulation is compromised, straight traction on the limb may reduce pressure on a blood vessel from a displaced bone end or remove a "kink" in the vessel from the angulated position of the limb. Traction should be applied gently, slowly, and in line with the limb; never should an attempt to forcibly reduce the fracture be performed. Documenting circulation before and after this maneuver is critical information for the treating emergency department to have. Also, transportation to the hospital should not be delayed in order to try and get circulation to return while the athlete is on the field. Splinting is then performed with the traction being held; this will improve the chances the limb will remain "straight" after splint application.

Compartment syndrome can occur following fracture due to rapid swelling in the closed compartments of the leg and forearm. The lower leg (below the knee) and forearm (elbow to hand) are the most common locations where a compartment syndrome can develop; however, it should never be assumed it cannot occur anywhere else (ie, thigh, foot, hand). The classic signs of compartment syndrome are remembered as the "5 Ps": pain, pallor (whiteness), paresthesia (numbness or tingling), pulselessness, and paralysis.

In general, symptoms should never get beyond pain because this is the first to occur. Severe damage may have already occurred to the limb once symptoms progress to the other symptoms. The pain with compartment syndrome is usually severe, unresponsive to splinting and medication, and out of proportion to what one might expect to see from an injury. Bandages or compression wraps can make symptoms worse and should be loosened; this alone sometimes relieves the pain. If the loosening of the bandage or wrap relieves the pain, it is likely that a full blown compartment syndrome has not yet occurred. If there is any question, immediate transfer to the hospital is required. Surgery is usually the only treatment for this syndrome.

Dislocations

A dislocation is the most severe form of ligament and/or joint capsule injury. The normal relationship between the 2 bones forming the joint is lost; basically, the "ball is out of the socket."

EVALUATION

Dislocations can occur at any joint. There is an obvious injury in most cases and the individual may have heard a "pop" or felt the joint "slide" out of place. Pain is usually severe and motion is virtually impossible.

Attempts to passively range the joint are unsuccessful; there is a block to motion from the abnormal relationship of the 2 ends of the joint to one another. The ends are overlapping, creating a block to motion. The athlete is typically holding the injured limb to protect him- or herself from painful attempts at moving the joint (commonly known as "splinting"). A deformity is usually more obvious with a superficial joint, such as the fingers.

As with any extremity injury, careful evaluation of nerve function below the injury level is critical. Document all nerve function prior to any attempts at reducing the joint. Vascular status should similarly be evaluated and documented. The signs of nerve and vascular injury, as noted above for fractures, apply to dislocations as well.

Initial Treatment

A trained member of the medical team can attempt a gentle reduction or "popping" the joint back in place. Forceful attempts to reduce the joint should never be attempted because there can be a tendon, ligament, or piece of bone trapped in the joint, preventing reduction. Also, a forceful reduction can cause a fracture or make an associated fracture worse.

If the initial reduction attempt is successful, there will usually be a much more fluid motion to the joint and the athlete will be nearly pain free. In this scenario, the athlete can be placed in a splint or immobilizer (depending on the joint involved) and sent for x-rays that day or evening. It is important to always get x-rays to rule out a fracture and ensure there has been an adequate reduction. Often, an athlete can tell if the joint is reduced or not; when told by an individual that the joint is "not in," this should be taken seriously.

In the event that a trained and qualified person to reduce the joint is not available, the athlete should be transported to the local emergency room for x-rays and reduction there. Also, any signs of nerve or vascular injury require immediate transfer to the hospital, even if a successful reduction has been performed.

Emergencies

As with fractures, any open dislocations require immediate attention. Also, any nerve or vascular injuries should be considered emergencies. As stated above, a joint that cannot be reduced should also be considered an emergency.

Principles of Splinting

Splinting of fractures, dislocations, or other extremity injuries has a number of benefits and should be included in the initial emergency management. Splinting benefits the injured athlete in the following ways:

- Reduces pain and swelling
- Prevents further blood vessel and nerve injury from sharp fracture ends
- Prevents sharp fracture ends from piercing the skin (turning a closed fracture to an open one)
- Decreases further contamination of open wounds

GENERAL PRINCIPLES

Sports emergency care personnel should follow these guidelines whenever splinting a fracture or dislocation:

- Remove clothing around the suspected injury to make sure there are no open wounds or deformities.
- Check pulse and nerve function below level of injury prior to splinting.
- Cover wounds with sterile dressing as noted previously (see Table 11-1).
- Splint should immobilize above and below area of injury.
- Pad splint well to avoid pressure points from rigid splints.
- Hold extremity immobile until splint hardens in desired position.
- If a deformity cannot be "straightened" by gentle, continuous traction, splint the limb in the position of deformity.

MATERIALS

There are a variety of options when it comes to splinting and all have their own pros and cons. It is beyond the scope of this chapter to critically analyze each type of splint, but general principles will be addressed. Splints come in plaster, fiberglass, moldable thermoplastic material, metal (usually aluminum for easy molding), and pneumatic (air splints). In addition, there are numerous preshaped splints; however, the "do-it-yourself" molding types usually are the most versatile. The advantage of prefabricated splints is they do not require water or heat to work. In general, most items can be used for a variety of extremity and joint injuries. The athletic trainer should sample several different splints and splinting materials to decide which he or she is most comfortable using. Proper preparation before an injury occurs will decrease the chance the trainer is on the field with an emergency and does not have the proper tools. What is presented here is an example of different, available materials and is by no means all-inclusive. See Table 11-2 for some basic points on material types. Figure 11-4 shows examples of different materials commonly used.

The sports emergency care team should keep several different types and sizes of splinting material on hand. Cast padding of various sizes should be on hand for use when using plaster or fiberglass splints. Padding will decrease pressure from the splint and protect the skin. The padding, like splinting material, comes in a variety of sizes (typically 1 inch to 6 inches) in order to accommodate most joints and extremities. A bucket to fill with water is useful as well because plaster and fiberglass need to be wet in order to shape and to set or harden. A good pair of scissors to cut the material is essential as well. Gloves should be used when utilizing plaster and especially fiberglass to protect the user's hands. Several sizes of elastic bandages are required to hold the splint in place.

Table 11-2

SPLINTING MATERIALS

Splint Material	Padding Required	Water Required	Reusable	Heat Required
Plaster	Yes	Yes	No	No
Fiberglass	Yes	Yes	No	No
Aluminum	No	No	Often	No
Plastic	Sometimes	Sometimes	Yes	Yes
Pneumatic	No	No	Yes	No

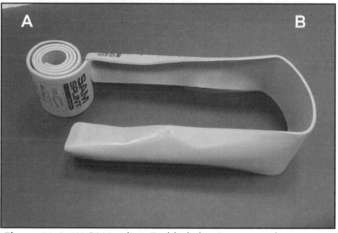

Figure 11-4. (A) SAM splint. Padded aluminum core for easy use and molding. (B) Different view of SAM splint.

COMPLICATIONS OF SPLINTING

The major complication of splinting is a compartment syndrome. This is usually secondary to the cast padding or elastic bandage being wrapped too tightly or the application of a circumferential cast being applied too tightly. It is rarely necessary to apply a circumferential cast in the field, so this should not be a problem. As noted earlier, pain that is severe or out of proportion to what is expected is the first sign of an impending compartment syndrome. When an athlete complains of this kind of pain or tightness, it should raise a

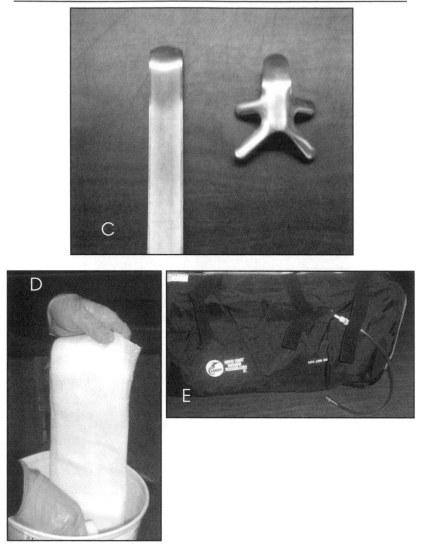

Figure 11-4. (C) Aluminum splints for small joint (finger) splinting. Padded and can be cut to fit better. Also, easily molded and can be secured with tape or elastic bandage. (D) Fiberglass material. Fiberglass, like plaster, requires water to harden or "set." Comes in variety of sizes from 1 inch to 6 inches, can literally be used to splint any joint or extremity. (E) Pneumatic splint. This is a Cramer Rapid Form Vacuum Immobilizer (Cramer Products Inc, Gardner, Kan).

red flag. Simply loosening the elastic wrap will usually rapidly relieve the pain (within minutes). Avoiding the placement of cast padding circumferentially around the injured extremity will help to avoid this complication as well.

Splinting by Extremity

HAND AND WRIST

Prefabricated splints are easy to use and versatile for the majority of hand and finger injuries. They can often be used as protection and allow for functional return to athletic competition depending on the sport and the severity of the injury. Figure 11-5 shows examples of splints applied to the hand and wrist. The reader should realize that any plaster or fiberglass splint could be fashioned to work in the same way. Usually, the splint is applied to the volar (palm side) of the hand for hand and wrist injuries. The splint is applied to the hand and wrist area and an elastic bandage is wrapped around the splint to hold it in place. When making a fresh splint from plaster or fiberglass, be careful to use enough padding to avoid pressure points and heat injury while the material hardens.

Splints such as the aluminum types shown in Figure 11-4C are good for isolated finger injuries. These finger splints are typically placed on the dorsal (opposite palm side) for finger splinting. This allows for comfort and possible continued use of the hand while the splint is worn.

FOREARM AND ELBOW

It is often helpful to have the athlete lie down and an assistant hold his or her fingers for support. These splints need to include the elbow joint to provide the most stability and comfort. This type of splint is commonly referred to as a sugar-tong splint. A SAM splint is easy to use and easily molded for this application. In addition, it is reusable. However, any of these splints can be made out of simple plaster and/or fiberglass. Figure 11-6 shows an example of SAM splint application for a forearm injury. As shown in this example, including the hand improves comfort for forearm/elbow injuries because the muscles that move the wrist cross the elbow and insert or originate from the humerus.

Another useful splint for injuries to the forearm and elbow is the posterior splint. Again, this can be made of plaster, fiberglass, or from SAM splinting material. See Figure 11-7 for an example of a posterior splint application utilizing plaster as the material. The cast padding is laid out to the appropriate length (based on the individual's arm length); the plaster is then laid out to be slightly smaller length than the padding. Usually 8 layers of plaster are utilized; too few layers make the splint weak and too many layers can increase

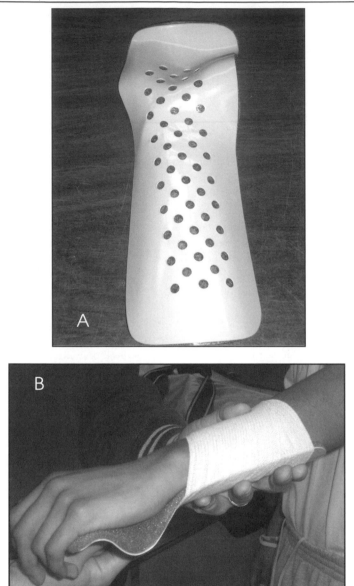

Figures 11-5. Wrist splint application.

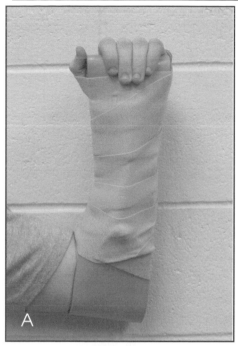

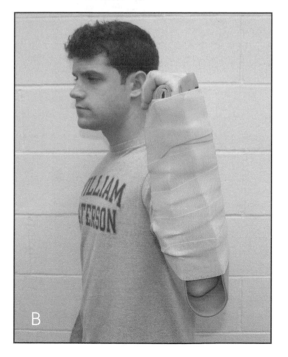

Figures 11-6. Immobilization of the forearm using a SAM splint.

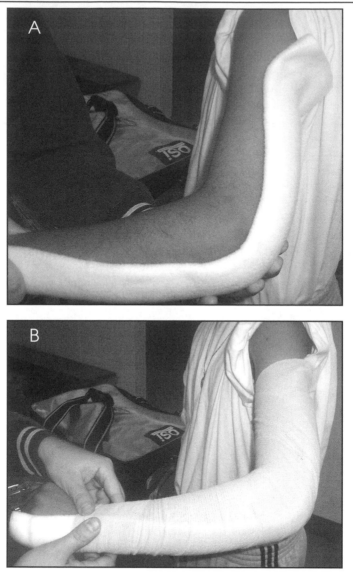

Figure 11-7. Elbow immobilization.

the risk of thermal injury. The plaster is placed in water and then back onto the padding; an additional layer of padding is placed on top, covering the plaster on both sides. The splint is held in place and wrapped with an elastic bandage.

ARM

Splinting suspected humerus fractures is basically the same as for elbow and forearm injuries, but the splint wraps around the elbow and the arm above. Also, a simple sling may be sufficient if no splinting material is available or for comfort to hold the arm while in a splint. A sling is usually all that is required for shoulder injuries because splinting the shoulder is difficult. The posterior splint (see Figure 11-7) can be used for this as well.

THIGH AND KNEE

Immobilizing the thigh can be difficult. In this scenario, a pneumatic splint may be the best splint to provide stability to a suspected femur fracture. Also, ligament sprains and fractures of the knee are well immobilized in these splints. If a deformity exists, it is helpful to have an assistant pull gentle traction from the foot to "straighten" the leg. Holding the leg in this position prior to applying the pneumatic brace or splint will increase the chances that the deformity will not return while in transport to the hospital. Figure 11-8 shows a Cramer Rapid Form Immobilizer being placed on a knee.

LEG, ANKLE, AND FOOT

There are a variety of ways to splint this area. The vacuum splint in Figure 11-8 can work well for leg or tibia injuries or the sugar-tong splint in Figure 11-6 can easily be made for a leg or ankle injury. The SAM splint, fiberglass, or plaster can all be used to make the splint. The posterior splint is simple and useful as well. This is basically the same as the splint shown in Figure 11-7 but adapted for the leg. A posterior leg splint utilizing fiberglass is shown in Figure 11-9. When applying a splint to the leg, the ankle should be held as close to neutral or a 90-degree angle as possible, as shown in Figure 11-9.

Open Wounds

An open wound is an injury in which the skin is interrupted, or broken, exposing the tissue underneath. The interruption can come from the outside such as with a laceration or from the inside such as when a fractured bone end tears outward through the skin. Sports emergency care personnel should be sure to observe body substance isolation and utilize personal protective equipment before treating any athlete with an open wound (Table 11-3).

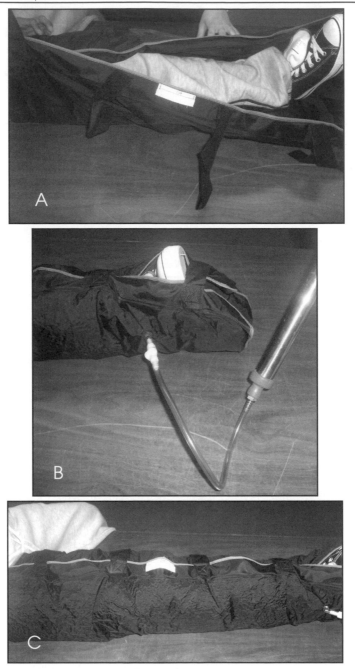

Figure 11-8. Vacuum splint application.

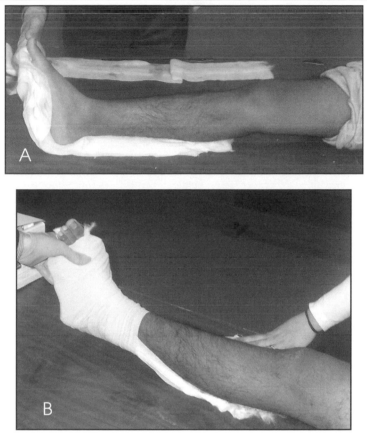

Figure 11-9. Splint application to the ankle and lower leg.

TYPES OF OPEN WOUNDS

Abrasions and Lacerations

The classification of abrasions includes simple scrapes and scratches in which the outer layer of the skin is damaged but all layers are not penetrated. "Road rash," "mat burn," "floor burn," and skinned knees and elbows are examples of abrasions. There may be no detectable bleeding or only a minor ooze of blood from the capillary beds. The patient may be experiencing great pain, even if the injury is minor. The opportunity for infection is great because of dirt or other substances ground into the skin.

A laceration is a cut that can be either smooth (resembling an incision) or jagged. This type of wound is often caused by an object with a sharp edge such

---

Table 11-3

OPEN WOUND GENERAL TREATMENT GUIDELINES

These guidelines are general guidelines; see each specific type of wound for more detailed guidelines.

* Isolate the body substance.
* Expose the wound.
* Clean the wound surface. Simply remove large pieces of debris with a sterile dressing.
* Control the bleeding. Start with direct pressure or direct pressure and elevation. When necessary, employ pressure. (A tourniquet is only to be used as a last resort!)
* Treat for shock in cases of more serious wounds.
* Wrap with a sterile dressing when available.
* Bandage the dressing in place when bleeding has been controlled.
* Check distal pulses.

---

as a piece of sharp metal or broken glass. However, a laceration can also result from a severe blow or impact with a blunt object (ie, being punched or being struck by a hockey puck or ball). It may be difficult to determine the extent of damage in lacerations with rough edges because the damaged flaps of skin may hide damage to the underlying tissues. Obviously, deeper wounds will produce significant bleeding. However, bleeding may be partially controlled in some wounds by the natural retraction and constriction of the damaged blood vessels.

The first step in treating abrasions and lacerations is to reduce wound contamination. Bleeding from a large or deep laceration may be difficult to control. Applying direct pressure over the wound should always be the first method of bleeding control. Using direct pressure, followed by the application of a dressing and a pressure bandage, can control most wounds. In cases of more severe bleeding, an air-inflated splint or blood pressure cuff can be useful in the management of bleeding; however, great care must be taken to prevent further injury or complications that may arise from overinflation of the splint or cuff. A wound closure such as a butterfly-type bandage or Steri-Strips (3M, St. Paul, Minn) can help keep wound ends together temporarily in severe lacerations. Pulses and motor and sensory functions should be checked distal to the injury. In cases when bleeding from lacerations cannot be controlled with the above mentioned treatment, the patient may require sutures, plastic surgery, and/or a tetanus shot, thus referral to a physician or hospital is required.

Puncture Wounds

Puncture wounds can be caused by objects that go undetected on playing fields or courts, such as nails, knives, splinters, or other sharp objects. The threat of contamination in a puncture wound is significant. A penetrating puncture wound can be shallow or deep. A perforating puncture wound has both an entrance wound and an exit wound. These wounds are not very common in sports as the most common example is a gunshot wound.

Use caution when treating puncture wounds. An object that appears to be embedded only in the skin may actually go all the way to the bone. In such cases, it is possible that the patient may not have serious pain due to either shock or damage to the nerves. Even an apparently moderate puncture wound may cause extensive internal injury with serious internal bleeding. What appears at first to be a simple, shallow puncture wound may be only part of a bigger, more severe injury. There also could be an exit wound that requires immediate care, so always be sure to evaluate for one.

A puncture wound may contain an impaled object. In sports, the object can be a piece of glass, a post, a sharp piece of metal, a javelin, or possibly even a wooden stick from a broken bat piercing any part of the body. Even though it is rare, the sports emergency care personnel may be confronted with a case where the impaled object is too long to make even emergency transport possible without shortening the object (ie, a javelin). In such cases, the sports emergency care personnel team must work together to determine what is the best direction to move in for the athlete/patient. In most cases, someone must hold the object, keeping it very stable, while it is gently sawed to the desired length. A fine-toothed saw with a rigid blade support should be used.

Never remove an impaled object. Doing so could cause further injury. The object may play a role in controlling the bleeding by acting as a barrier against severed blood vessels. Removal of the object may cause massive bleeding as well as further injury to nerves, muscles, and other soft tissues. Proceed as follows:

- Expose the wound area.
- Control bleeding with direct pressure, if possible.
- While the sports emergency care team stabilizes the object and controls bleeding, have another trained sports medicine team member place several layers of bulky dressing around the injury so that the dressing surrounds the object on all sides. Continue placing dressings, pads, and other bulky materials around the wound until the object is as secure as possible. Once bandaged in place, the dressing will stabilize the object and exert downward pressure on the bleeding vessels.
- Secure the dressings in place.
- Care for shock.

- Position the patient to ensure minimal stress.

- Transport the patient to a medical facility as soon as possible.

Impaled objects in the cheek may be removed if they pose a threat to the airway. Remove the object by gently pulling it out in the direction that it entered the cheek. If this cannot be done easily, leave the object in place. Do not twist the object. If the second end of the object is impaled into a deeper structure, inhibiting you from seeing the second end, stabilize the object. Be prepared to control bleeding at the wound site from both inside and outside the mouth.

Treatment of an impaled object in the eye includes stabilizing the object using rolls of gauze or similar material. Stabilize the object on both sides. Place a cover over the uninjured eye to help reduce sympathetic eye movement.

Avulsion Wounds

Flaps of skin and tissues are torn loose or pulled off completely in an avulsion wound. When the tip of the nose is cut or torn off, this is an avulsion. The same applies to the external ear. An eye pulled out from its socket (extruded) is a form of an avulsion. The term avulsed is used in reporting the wound as in "avulsed eye" or an "avulsed ear." When tissue is avulsed, it is cut off from its oxygen supply and will die soon. In sports, the most common avulsions are a tooth avulsion, finger avulsion (in weight lifting), and ear avulsion.

Emergency care for avulsions is similar to that of other open wounds. Apply direct pressure using a sterile dressing. If the avulsed skin becomes detached, save the avulsed part by wrapping it in a dry sterile gauze dressing secured in place by self-adherent roller bandage. Then place it in a plastic bag and send it to the hospital along with the athlete. Make sure to label the avulsed part with the following information: name of body part (and side), the patient's name and date, and the time the part was wrapped and bagged. The record should show the approximate time of the avulsion. Keep the part as cool as possible, without freezing it, by placing it in a cooler or any other available container so that it is on top of a cold pack or a sealed bag of ice. DO NOT USE DRY ICE! Do not immerse the avulsed part in ice, cooled water, or saline. Label the container the same as the label used for the saved part.

Amputations

Amputations, although rare in sports, can occur. An amputation is when the fingers, toes, hands, feet, or limbs are completely severed from the body. Jagged skin and bone edges may be present, and there may be massive bleeding. Often, blood vessels retract, which limits bleeding from the wound site.

Treatment of amputations includes applying a pressure dressing over the distal edge of the amputation site. Pressure points may also be used to control the bleeding. A tourniquet should not be applied unless other methods used to control bleeding have failed. Wrap the amputated part in a sterile dressing and place it in a plastic bag. Place the bag in a cooler with ice. Do not bury the amputated part in the ice. Do not use dry ice to cool the part!

Conclusion

Management of fractures and dislocations on the field requires the careful inspection of the involved extremity, removing the athlete from further harm, splinting the injured extremity to protect the limb and provide comfort, then appropriate transfer to an emergency care center or hospital. Careful extremity assessment for open wounds, nerve or vascular injury, and deformity will avoid undue delays in transfer for appropriate care and give the athlete the best chance of avoiding complications from their injuries.

Bibliography

Campbell JE. *Basic Trauma Life Support for the EMT-B and the First Responder.* Upper Saddle River, NJ: Pearson Prentice Hall; 2004.

Greene WB, ed. *Essentials of Musculoskeletal Care.* 2nd ed. Rosemont, Ill: American Academy of Orthopedic Surgeons; 2001.

Jenkins DB. *Organs and Organ Systems.* 8th ed. Philadelphia: WB Saunders Company; 2002.

Limmer D, O'Keefe MF, Grant HD, Murray RH, Bergeron JD. *Emergency Care.* Upper Saddle River, NJ: Brady/Prentice Hall Health; 2001.

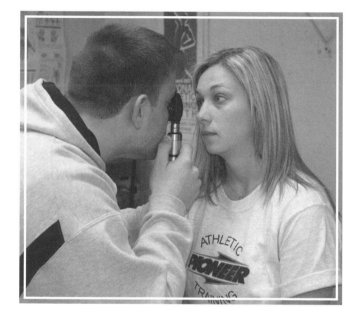

Chapter 12 *General Medical Emergencies*

John L. Davis, MS, ATC

When athletic trainers, coaches, and athletes think of injuries in athletics, they most often visualize the standard orthopedic problems that are most common in sports. When parents, administrators, the lay public, and other health care professionals think of injuries, they usually think of the more systemic, large-scale problems that call immediate attention to the field due to the need for quick response and transportation via an ambulance. Athletic trainers and other sports emergency care providers will need to work as a team to evaluate and provide quality and efficient emergency care to the injured athlete. The sports emergency care team needs to be well educated, practiced, and prepared for recognition and treatment of such conditions as shock, environmental emergencies (cold exposure and heat disorders), and other general medical conditions such as asthma, diabetes, and mononucleosis.

Shock: Orientation to Anatomy and Physiology

In many respects, the essence of what an athletic trainer does every day is to manage the blood flow of the athletes he or she treats. To treat an athlete for acute swelling, we put ice on a body part to slow blood flow. To improve blood flow after the initial swelling has stopped, we put heat on a body part to increase blood flow or use active exercise to get the blood flowing.

The body is an amazing machine and it has the unique ability to adapt to different conditions, stresses, injuries, or illnesses. A simple understanding of the body's response to stress (injury) and how it adapts to intrinsic and extrinsic forces via changes in blood flow will help the sports emergency care provider tend to injured athletes more efficiently.

An explanation of the cardiovascular system starts with the idea that the system is made up of a container and its contents. The container is made of the muscular heart and the elastic vessels (arteries, veins, arterioles, venules, and capillaries). The contents of the system consist of the 12.6 pints (6 L) of blood that the average adult has circulating through the body daily. Each part of the body gets a regular supply of blood. Blood flowing through the system is the method through which the body maintains its normal temperature (98.6°F or 37°C) and transport oxygen (O_2) and nutrients to each part of the body while removing waste products and carbon dioxide (CO_2).

Shock

Shock is defined as a syndrome in which the peripheral flow of blood is insufficient to return enough blood to the heart for normal function. Shock is the body's attempt to prioritize and maintain the vital organs. The normal circulation of blood (perfusion) and O_2 to organs and tissues of the body is compromised (hypoperfusion) during shock, depressing the body's vital functions. Think of shock as a basic defensive mechanism of the body.

Some tissues in the body are more sensitive to a lack of O_2 than others. For instance, brain tissue ischemia occurs when the brain has been deprived of O_2 for as little as 4 minutes to 6 minutes. The heart muscle needs a constant supply of O_2, whereas the kidneys can survive 45 minutes without O_2 and skeletal muscles can last 2 hours.

Shock can occur as a result of many factors or stresses to the body. Every injury or medical condition to some extent causes a circulatory response and is influenced by the physical characteristics of the patient. Examples of some causative factors are trauma, drugs, poison, anoxia, hemorrhage, infection, dehydration, excessive heat, cold exposure, and choking or airway obstruction. The patient's age and general physical condition will go a long way in determining how severe a reaction the body exhibits.

There are many types of shock (Table 12-1), each caused by different factors. The body responds by creating a systemic shock in one of the following basic 3 ways: A pump failure occurs when the heart is damaged in some way, such as in a myocardial infarction resulting from coronary artery blockage. Pipe failure is caused when the blood vessels are injured in some way, such as when an athlete suffers a laceration or external bleeding associated with a compound fracture. Fluid failure is caused when there is a general vasodilation or widening of the peripheral blood vessels due to a toxic reaction in the blood caused by some infection. Septic shock is an example of fluid failure.

The body will always respond to an injury or illness in one of the following 3 ways:

1. Changing the flow of blood by speeding up or slowing the rate of the heart.

Table 12-1

TYPES OF SHOCK

Type	Description	Cause
Anaphylactic	Allergic reaction to an allergen	Pipe failure
Cardiogenic	Conditions affecting the heart	Pump failure
Hypovolemic	Blood loss from bleeding	Pump failure
Metabolic	Fluid loss from vomiting, diarrhea, and urination	Fluid failure
Neurogenic	Vasodilation of peripheral blood vessels due to neurological injury	Pipe failure
Psychogenic	Vasodilation of peripheral blood vessels due to psychological response	Pipe failure
Septic	Vasodilation of peripheral blood vessels and blood leaking out of the blood vessels due to infection/toxins	Fluid failure

2. Increasing (vasodilating) or decreasing (vasoconstricting) the size of the blood vessels locally or throughout the system.

3. Increasing or decreasing the amount of fluid content of blood in the system. (Blood has both a fluid [plasma] component and a solid [red and white blood cells and platelets] component.)

As stated previously, the sports emergency care provider must take these changes into consideration and respond to the signs and symptoms that the injured athlete's body presents.

HISTORY AND EXAMINATION

It is easy to understand how the body responds to an injury leading to shock if we follow a typical injury scenario and review how the body's vital signs and essential processes are affected. The vital signs are the signs and symptoms that you look for to give you clues to what is going on inside the body.

For example, an athlete suffers a compound fracture of his ankle playing soccer. The tibia and fibula are both fractured and the distal portion of the tibia is protruding through the skin. There is significant bleeding due to a lacerated artery.

- The heart responds initially to local bleeding by increasing the heart rate. (Rapid pulse)

- The athlete is also emotionally anxious, restless, and in severe pain due to the damage to the nervous system. (Restlessness, irritability, anxiety)
- As the bleeding continues, the blood volume will drop as more blood is lost. (Pulse becomes rapid and weak and may become difficult to find. Blood pressure subsequently decreases.)
- The body will try to take fluid from other parts of the body to allow the production of more blood and increase the fluid portion of blood. (Excessive thirst)
- The body is now working hard to try and fight the injury. The breathing rate increases because there is a higher demand for O_2 at the injury site and throughout the body.
- To control the flow of blood and focus on the injured area and the vital internal organs, the blood vessels will constrict in skin away from the injury. The skin will appear to be pale and cold to the touch. This will decrease the blood flow to uninjured areas while increasing it to areas under stress. In a further response the body will start to sweat heavily (diaphoresis), leaving the skin moist and clammy.
- Some tissues in the body may be without O_2 for a period of time, so the body at some point will try to get O_2 to those body parts by rebalancing or equalizing the blood flow through all its parts by pulling blood from the vital organs.
- The vital organs are now without proper O_2. (Further increasing breathing and pulse rate.)
- O_2 is the key to function throughout the body. The vital organs will start to function poorly without O_2 and the brain, the controlling mechanism, will begin to be affected. The athlete will get lightheaded or feel as though he or she is about to faint. The pupils may have a dull, vacant look. As the cascade of poor function continues, the athlete will become drowsy and he or she may become more restless. His level of consciousness will eventually suffer.
- The heart muscle itself, which has been working extremely hard, will finally be affected as it gets deprived of O_2 and blood due to the compromised circulation. The heart rate and pulse will become increasingly faster and more irregular as the heart fights to keep itself and the body alive. The pulse will no longer be detectable.

The body fought to compensate for the severe blood loss by constantly changing the flow of blood through the body. In this example, the cascade of physiological events unfortunately resulted in this athlete entering into a severe state of shock.

Table 12-2

SIGNS AND SYMPTOMS OF SHOCK

Vital Sign	Sign/Symptom
Heart rate	Decreasing (rapid then decreasing)
Pulse rate	Rapid, weak
Respiratory rate	Rapid and shallow
Skin color	Pale, blue, or gray
Skin temperature	Cool and moist (clammy)
Eyes	Dull, listless
Muscle function	Decreasing ability to control
Nausea/vomiting	Excessive thirst
Mental status	Lightheaded Restlessness, irritability, anxiety Drowsy, LOC

MANAGEMENT AND TREATMENT

Sports emergency care providers must use their skills, experience, and knowledge to fully assess and determine the required care and treatment of injured athletes. Table 12-2 describes the signs and symptoms an injured athlete may exhibit during shock. Care of an athlete suspected of having shock or potentially experiencing shock should include the following steps:

- Do no further harm. Do not move the athlete and create additional injury.
- Assess ABCx3.
- Maintain an open airway, watch breathing, and control bleeding.
- Elevate lower extremities 12 inches (as long as there is not an upper body injury).
- A patient suffering a heart attack may be more comfortable in a semi-reclining position.
- Maintain the athlete's body heat (use blankets above and below if necessary).
- Reassure and calm the athlete and try to have him or her rest comfortably.

- Treat trauma to the body such as fractures or bleeding.
- Document and monitor vital signs.
- Limit fluids and food.

By correctly recognizing the signs and symptoms of shock, an emergency care provider will be able to assist the body in making natural adaptations. Once the athlete arrives at a hospital, more definitive care can be given to treat the condition that precipitated shock. Transfusions may be necessary for someone who lost a significant amount of blood. A patient who suffers from a cardiac-related episode may be given medication to help the damaged heart. A patient who suffers from a dilated vascular system will receive medication to constrict the blood vessels. An athlete with an orthopedic injury, such as a fracture, will be splinted, casted, or surgically treated to correct the problem.

Environmental Emergencies

Not all sports emergencies are orthopedic in nature. Sometimes the emergency will be related to the environment in which the athlete participates. Heat exhaustion and heat stroke are 2 hot climate-related conditions. Cold exposure, frostbite, and frostnip occur in cold weather activities such as skiing. Altitude disorders such as altitude sickness and mountain sickness occur when people enjoy recreational activities at high altitudes. In any event, sports emergency care personnel must be aware of the unique injury potential in any activity, location, or climate in which they may be providing care.

Heat Disorders

Dehydration, or lack of fluid in the body, can manifest itself in several ways and create imbalances of fluid and electrolytes. There are 3 heat disorders that can affect an athlete. Heat cramps are the easiest to treat, heat exhaustion is more intense, and heat stroke is more severe and life threatening.

To fully understand heat disorders, one must have a basic understanding of heat regulation in the body. The body uses blood to cool itself and carry heat from its core organs to the peripheral skin vessels where heat can be released. The hypothalamus regulates body temperature. The impulses to increase body sweating and peripheral vasodilation result from temperature elevations in the hypothalamus. The normal body temperature is 98.6°F. The body generates heat to maintain an optimal internal environment. Heat is also created as a byproduct of muscle activity.

When necessary, heat is dissipated by varying the blood flow to the peripheral vessels in the skin. When the blood reaches vessels near the skin, heat will normally be released into the surrounding air, effectively cooling the skin and blood in the peripheral blood vessels. If the body is engaged in physical activity, is challenged by high temperatures, or a combination of both, the body

Table 12-3

HUMIDITY AND SWEATING CHART

Relative Humidity	Sweating Mechanism
60%	Working fairly well
70% to 75%	Evaporation, radiation, and respiration methods fail. Conduction and convection are most effective methods.
90%	Conduction is the only method working.

will generate more heat internally. This heat will be carried to the skin by blood and if the peripheral blood vessels are vasodilated, additional heat will be released. Heat loss occurs at the skin surface in 5 interrelated ways.

1. Convection: Air currents move across the skin, and heat is transferred to the cooler air around the body. This is similar to blowing on hot food to cool it down.

2. Conduction: Water or solid objects (ie, T-shirt) act as a wick to directly pull heat away from the body.

3. Radiation: Heat is released into the air. Think of baseboard heat in your house.

4. Evaporation: Sweat on the body is vaporized.

5. Respiration: Cool air taken into the lungs is warmed and heat is lost through this transfer.

Under normal conditions, 70% of body heat is dissipated by radiation and convection. As long as the temperature of the surrounding climate is below that of the body, heat will be released easily. When the temperature of surrounding air is equal to or above 98°F to 99°F, the only effective heat loss mechanisms are conduction and sweating (evaporation) (Table 12-3). When the surrounding humidity is high (close to 100%), the only means of heat loss will be conduction. An athlete will have to wipe the sweat off his or her body.

As heat and humidity increase and/or physical activity increases, body metabolism jumps dramatically. As stated previously, the body generates heat as a byproduct of muscle contraction as physical activity increases. Consequently, the body temperature increases. The brain and hypothalamus, via the CNS, will then increase the sweating mechanism and dilate the peripheral vessels to carry heat out of the body.

As heated blood reaches the skin via the dilated blood vessels, water and electrolytes such as sodium chloride, potassium, magnesium, and calcium are carried out of the skin via sweat. These minerals will either drip from the body, be wicked away via conduction into a shirt, or be wiped off with a towel.

Too much water and electrolyte loss will affect muscle physiology and the ability of the muscles to contract properly. Water is vital to body homeostasis, and a decrease will lead to a lower blood volume, lower cardiac output, and a decreased velocity of blood flow. The water, salt, and other electrolytes are responsible for maintaining the fluid balance in the intra- and extracellular areas. Salt (sodium chloride) in particular is important for maintaining osmotic pressure of the tissue cells. Osmotic pressure is created at the cell wall so the pressure inside and outside of the semipermeable membrane of the cell is equal. Calcium, sodium, and potassium are important for muscle contraction. An imbalance of water and the improper concentrations of salt, potassium, calcium, etc will lead to an impairment of the functioning of the muscles and vital body organs and systems.

As little as 3% of the total body weight lost in a day will lead to changes in judgment, weakness, and decreased muscular efficiency. A normal adult can only sweat about 1 qt/hour and only for a few hours before dehydration limits the output. As the activity increases in length or intensity, the amount of water sweated out will increase in salt concentration. As sweating increases, so does salt loss. Salt loss will vary in proportion to the fluid taken in. If the athlete drinks more, the salt concentration in the sweat on the skin will decrease. The athlete can change the amount he or she sweats by acclimatizing or getting conditioned to the hot, humid environment. The amount of salt lost varies with acclimatization and physical condition.

To summarize how the heat regulatory mechanisms in the hypothalamus and the body affect an athlete's blood flow, see the steps below:

- Blood goes to skin to release heat (peripheral vasodilatation).

- Less blood goes to the internal organs.

- The rates of perspiration and salt loss are increased.

- The rate of respiration is increased.

- The heart rate and stroke volume are increased.

- Salt concentration is increased as sweating continues.

- Efficient muscle activity due to loss of electrolytes and fatigue is decreased.

- More water is needed to balance the fluid loss from the body in general and the blood volume in particular. Water will be pulled from the internal organs such as the stomach and kidneys.

Types of Heat Disorders

Heat Cramps

- Definition: Muscle spasm or cramping due to fluid and/or salt loss. A cramp can be defined as a sudden involuntary movement or painful muscular contraction that does not relax due to an irritant or trauma.[1]

- Etiology: Heat cramps usually, but not always, are the first sign the athlete displays of dehydration. Normal contraction and relaxation of a muscle requires a balance of salt and water inside the muscle. There may be a localized loss of water and/or salt with heavy activity, and the muscle may spasm due to a decrease of the normal water and salt concentrations.

- History and Examination: This usually occurs early in the preseason conditioning phase. Cramping is caused by muscle fatigue, salt loss, and dehydration all working together. Cramping can affect any muscle, but most times shows up in the calf or gastric area due to the fact that most athletes are on their feet and the leg muscles will be working the hardest (Table 12-4). The abdomen, hamstring, and quadriceps muscles will also commonly cramp. In extreme cases of dehydration, the athlete can cramp in several muscle groups at the same time, indicating a more systemic or whole body response. Some athletes seem to be prone to heat cramps and may encounter them often and throughout the season.

- Management and Treatment: Initial treatment consists of resting and stretching the affected muscle. Massaging or kneading the muscle may also be effective. Obviously the sports emergency care provider would suggest the athlete increase fluid intake. In very persistent cases, the athletic trainer may try an ice massage on the affected muscle.

  The athlete's ability to play through the cramping will be determined by his or her physical condition, pain tolerance, the amount of time the cramping continued, and the ability to stop the cramping. The athletic trainer must be ready for the athlete to be sore and uncomfortable the next day due to the damage done to the muscle.

Heat Exhaustion

- Definition: Heat exhaustion, also known as "heat prostration," is the body's reaction to excessive heat and dehydration in which the sweating mechanism (Table 12-5) is working overtime and the athlete is sweating heavily, water and electrolytes are being lost, and the circulatory system is starting to struggle to keep pace with the need to cool the body. Body temperature is between 101°F and 104°F.

Table 12-4

SIGNS AND SYMPTOMS OF HEAT DISORDERS

Heat Cramps	Heat Exhaustion	Heat Stroke
Local muscle cramping	Profuse sweating	No sweating
Local skin moist	Cool, clammy skin	Hot, dry skin
Body temp is normal	Body temp is 101°F to 104°F	Body temp is above 105°F
	Pale, ashen skin	Red, flushed skin
	Excessive thirst	Thirsty if conscious
	Weak and rapid pulse	Weak and rapid pulse
	Dizzy, lightheaded	Loss of consciousness
	Nausea, vomiting	Nausea, vomiting
	Headaches	Increased heart and respiration
	Loss of muscle coordination	Mental confusion, disoriented
		Convulsions

Table 12-5

SWEATING FACTS

* Amount of water normally in adult male body is 42 L.
* 28 L are inside cells and 14 L are outside the cells (3 L of blood).
* Approximately 2 million sweat glands in the skin.
* Average sedentary adult takes in 2.5 L of water/day.
* Average runner needs additional 1.5 L to 2 L of water/hr of active sweating.
* Average runner in competition needs 2 L/hr to 4 L/hr of water.
* Athletes can lose 2 L to 8 L of water in 24 hours.
* Average person loses 2 g of salt in each liter of sweat.
* Average American takes in 5 g to 10 g of salt/day.
* Average American only needs 1 g to 3 g/day.
* With heavy activity, athlete can lose 5 L to 6 L of sweat in one event, which equals 2 lbs to 10 lbs of weight loss.
* As little as 1% to 2% of total body weight loss in a day leads to muscular inefficiency.

- Etiology: Heat exhaustion is more severe than heat cramps and is thought of as the second step or phase of heat disorders. Heat cramps may or may not precede heat exhaustion. Heat cramps may or may not occur at the same time. In this phase of heat syndrome complex, the body's cooling or sweating mechanism is barely keeping up with the need to get rid of internal heat. There is an inefficient cardiovascular response to stress of the environmental heat and humidity. The athlete's body will be working hard at exercise while also trying to cool itself. The muscles, brain, and other internal organs will demand increased blood flow during exercise, while more blood is needed by the skin and peripheral circulatory system to radiate heat away from the skin and cool the body. Water is being lost via sweat, so the fluid volume in both the body and blood is dropping. The body is simultaneously fighting 2 battles: progressive peripheral vascular collapse and mild hypovolemic shock (see Table 12-1).

- History and Examination: This syndrome usually occurs in the pre-season while the athlete is trying to acclimatize. In most cases, the athlete will be in poor shape during preseason training and will not handle the stress of the heavy activity. Many times the athlete affected will be an overweight, poorly conditioned, new member of the team who may not have understood the need to get in shape before the preseason activity started. Occasionally, the athletic trainer may run into a highly motivated, well-conditioned athlete who develops heat exhaustion because he or she worked so hard during 2-a-day practices that he or she does not recover well enough during the rest periods.

  Signs and symptoms of heat exhaustion (see Table 12-4) are as follows: profuse sweating; extreme thirst; pale, moist skin; slightly elevated skin temperature; weak and rapid pulse; dizziness and lightheadedness; chills; loss of coordination; nausea, vomiting, diarrhea; stomach cramps; and headaches.

- Management and Treatment: This athlete needs to be removed from activity and cooled immediately. Take the athlete to a shaded area or inside an air-conditioned room. Remove all excess clothing, keeping in mind the modesty of the athlete. Cool the athlete by placing ice or cool towels at the locations on the body where the blood passes close to the surface (ie, in the armpits, behind the neck, behind the knees, in the groin area, and on the forehead). Elevate the athlete's legs 12 inches to improve circulatory return to the heart. Spray the body with cold water. Use electric fans or fan the athlete with a towel. If the athlete is not nauseated or vomiting, give him or her cool water or an electrolyte drink to help cool the body from the inside out. In some athletic locations, you may be able to give intravenous fluid to speed the cooling and rehydration process. The athlete must be transported to a hospital for further evaluation, rehydration, and treatment.

Heat Stroke

- Definition: Heat stroke, which is the most severe heat syndrome, occurs when the body can no longer adequately cool itself, and the internal body temperature rises to a level that can cause the brain and internal organs to shut down. Heat stroke is a medical emergency and can result in death if not treated promptly. The body is literally overheating because the sweating mechanism has shut down to avoid further dehydration. Body temperature is above 105°F.

- Etiology: Heat stroke is a true medical emergency and must be acknowledged and treated as such. In this final stage of the heat syndrome complex, the body's cooling or sweating mechanism has failed to get rid of internal heat. The cardiovascular response to stress of the environmental heat and humidity has been overwhelmed. The athlete's blood volume will be very low due to the water lost and blood flow will be very poor. The body has lost the battle and is in full-blown peripheral vascular collapse or hypovolemic shock (see Table 12-1).

- History and Examination: This medical emergency occurs in hot, humid environments, usually during the preseason. There has been intense activity and little time to acclimatize. The athlete is probably in poor physical condition at the start of the preseason. Most heat stroke athletes are overweight and poorly conditioned.

Signs and symptoms of heat stroke (see Table 12-4) are as follows:

- No sweating
- Extreme thirst
- Hot, red, dry skin
- Elevated skin temperature
- Rapid and weak pulse
- Dizziness and lightheadedness, weakness, loss of coordination
- Convulsions
- Nausea, vomiting, diarrhea, stomach cramps
- Headaches
- Decreased blood pressure, increased heart rate; increased respiratory rate
- There may be a change in consciousness, and the athlete may be irritable, confused, hysterical, emotionally unstable, disorientated, or unconscious and in a coma

Table 12-6

CONDITIONING STANDARDS FOR HIGH HUMIDITY

Temperature	Humidity	Procedure
80°F to 90°F	Under 70%	Watch heavier athletes
80°F to 90°F	Over 70%	Frequent rest periods, change wet
90°F to 100°F	Under 70%	shirts. Monitor all athletes
90°F to 100°F Over 100°F	Over 70%	Consider changing practice time or altering practice length, intensity.

- Management and Treatment: Athletes in heat stroke need to be cooled immediately. Immediate whole-body cooling via cold water immersion is the best treatment and should start ASAP. If cold water immersion is not possible, the athlete can be cooled as was discussed in heat exhaustion. Assuming there is an appropriate sports emergency care team on site, the athlete should be cooled first. Transportation can occur after cooling. Take care to continually monitor the athlete's vital signs. If onsite cooling is not possible due to complications or lack of equipment, the athlete must be transported immediately. Intravenous saline should be introduced if possible. Be prepared to take core rectal temperatures to check the actual internal temperature. Core temperatures must be reduced to 101°F to 102°F. The athlete must be transported to a hospital for further evaluation, rehydration, and treatment.

- Special Considerations/Prevention: The best way to treat heat disorders or heat syndromes is to prevent them (Table 12-6). Heat cramps may be considered a regular and common injury that many athletes will suffer at some time. Heat exhaustion and heat stroke are mostly preventable occurrences. With proper preparation, athletes should be able to avoid these serious disorders. Simple methods to help prepare the athlete and the athletic trainer are easily established:

  ❖ Athletes need to acclimatize to their competitive environment before they arrive for preseason practice.

  ❖ Pre-hydrate. Drink before practice starts and throughout the day.

  ❖ Take regular water breaks.

❖   Encourage athletes to drink beyond their thirst. Drinking to thirst only restores about half of the fluid needed and will not satisfy the dehydrated water needs. Humans are the only mammals that do not drink to fully replenish the fluids needs of the body.

❖   Be sure athletes rehydrate between practices and replenish their water needs.

❖   Use available shade before and during practice when possible.

❖   Avoid caffeine, excessive protein, alcohol, and foods that make the athlete urinate.

❖   Monitor medications for adverse reactions.

❖   Be aware of proper diet and nutritional needs.

❖   Wear proper clothing (ie, loose, white, cotton or new fabrics that act as a wick).

❖   Listen to local weather forecasts and adjust practices accordingly.

❖   Avoid mid-day practices if possible. Try to practice early in the morning or in the early evening.

Most current weather forecasts in the warm summer months include a discussion of the heat index. The index is a combination of air temperature and relative humidity used to determine an apparent temperature (how hot it actually feels). Be sure to make use of these forecasts and be aware of the heat index because it can be used to alter daily practices. Refer to Table 12-7 for a review of the effects of the heat index on physical activity.

COLD EXPOSURE

Humans are basically semitropical creatures and the body is a heat-generating machine. We do not tolerate cold well and have a limited capability to protect ourselves from the dangers of prolonged low temperatures. We have learned to adapt to cold climates. As discussed in the previous section on heat disorders, the enzyme systems of the body work best when the normal body temperature of 98.6°F is maintained. If the core temperature of the body is reduced or compromised by 1 degree to 2 degrees, the body will not function 100% effectively.

When considering thermoregulation, the body should be considered in 2 parts: the core (brain, heart, lungs, and vital abdominal organs) and the shell (skin, muscles, and extremities). When the body gets cold, it attempts to correct the problem by increasing internal heat production. The first mechanism the body uses to fight the cold is to create muscular activity through shivering. If the shivering is not enough, hypothermic victims will instinctively start to create more movement by rocking back and forth, swinging arms, walking,

Table 12-7

EFFECTS OF THE HEAT INDEX

Temperature	Notes
80°F to 90°F	Caution—fatigue is possible with prolonged exposure and activity
90°F to 105°F	Extreme caution—heat cramps and heat exhaustion possible
105°F to 130°F	Danger—heat cramps and exhaustion likely, heat stroke possible
Over 130°F	Extreme danger—heat stroke likely with prolonged exposure

Reprinted from National Weather Service.

etc. This movement will help increase the body's metabolic rate to increase the heat production. To complement these attempts to increase the heat production and core temperature, the body will limit the heat loss via the skin by vasoconstriction of the peripheral blood vessels. In summary, the body will fight the cold climate by reducing the heat lost via conduction, convection, respiration, evaporation, and radiation and also by increasing the internal production of heat by initiating muscle contraction.

Types of Cold Exposure Injuries

Cold or freezing temperatures affect the extremities and exposed body parts most often. The fingers, toes, ears, and nose are most commonly affected and are obviously located at the end of the circulatory system and far from the heart. They are subject to rapid heat loss due to their location. The depth and extent of a cold exposure injury will be determined by the intensity of the cold, duration of exposure, and the wind velocity.

Frostnip

- Definition: Cooling or freezing of the cells at the tips of the ears, nose, cheeks, chin, fingers, and toes.
- Etiology: Frostnip is usually, but not always, the first sign the athlete displays of a cold exposure injury.
- History and Examination: This injury will manifest itself as red, swollen, painful skin and may turn white after prolonged exposure (Table 12-8).

Table 12-8

SIGNS AND SYMPTOMS OF COLD EXPOSURE INJURIES

Frostnip	Frostbite	Hypothermia
Tips of finger, toes, and ears	Fingers, toes, ears, nose	General body cooling
Skin may appear red (initially) or white	White or waxy	General paleness
Skin cool to touch	Cold to touch	Cold to touch
	Numbness	Numbness and weakness
	Tingling/pins and needles	Shivering
		Glassy stare, confusion
		Slow pulse and respirations
		Decreasing consciousness

- Management and Treatment: The athlete needs to warm the affected body part by putting the fingers in the armpit, blowing on the hand, or placing the hands on the affected part and allowing the hands to provide added warmth to block the cold. There normally is no tissue damage and the body part will return to normal shortly.

Frostbite

- Definition: Frostbite is defined as a freezing of the skin and flesh due to cold exposure.

- Etiology: Frostbite can be deep or superficial, but usually affects the skin and underlying tissue only. Cells are composed of mostly water and will get cold and eventually freeze when exposed to a cold environment for a prolonged period of time. Ice crystals will form and damage and destroy the affected cells.

- History and Examination: The skin will appear white and waxy and is cold and firm to the touch (see Table 12-8). The underlying tissue continues to be soft and resilient. Numbness and tingling will occur. With prolonged exposure, the capillaries will be damaged, plasma will leak out of the blood, and the deeper tissue will be affected. Blisters may form.

- Management and Treatment: Athletes with frostbite should be taken to a hospital for further evaluation. The skin needs to be rewarmed or thawed as soon as possible. Move the athlete to a warm environment. Use blankets or coats to keep the victim warm. If there is a chance the body part might refreeze, do not start to rewarm the body part until it can stay warm. Do not rub or massage the body part because doing so will damage the tissues further. Warm water baths (100°F to 105°F) can be used, but make sure the water is not too hot. Warm drinks can also help to raise the core temperature and stimulate increased blood flow. Handle the injured part gently and bandage it with dry sterile dressings. If fingers and/or toes are affected, keep them separated with gauze.

Hypothermia

- Etiology: Hypothermia is general cooling of the entire body. It can occur at temperatures above freezing if there is prolonged exposure to low or rapidly dropping temperatures, as affects many homeless people. As the condition continues, an abnormal heart rhythm may develop due to decreased core temperature and thickening of the blood, making circulation difficult. Alcohol, drugs, smoking, hunger, age, fatigue, physical condition, and level of exertion can aggravate hypothermia. Full or partial submersion in cold water, such as a lake or creek, will intensify and speed up the body's reaction to the cold environment.

- History and Examination: In most cases, shivering will be extensive, although shivering usually ceases in severe cases of hypothermia (body temperature below 86°F) (see Table 12-8). Numbness and weakness will occur. The athlete will have a glassy stare and may display difficulty speaking. Motor functions will be more difficult and the athlete will appear clumsy and slow. The pulse rate and respiration rate will decrease. There may be mental confusion, impaired judgment, and decreasing consciousness. Areas of frostbite may or may not be present.

- Management and Treatment: Gently move the athlete to a warm location and monitor vitals signs. Wet clothing must be removed and dry blankets or clothing should be used to prevent additional heat loss. Warm fluids should be given if the athlete is conscious. Warm the blood as quickly as possible by placing hot packs at the pressure points. Be ready to treat for shock and treat the athlete for cardiac arrhythmias.

- Special Considerations: As with heat disorders, the best way to treat cold injuries is to prevent them. Athletes usually have more difficulty acclimatizing to the cold than they do to the heat. Sports emergency care personnel must be aware of the daily weather forecast to try and plan for and prevent these injuries. Anticipate weather changes, and be prepared for athletes to be underprepared. Athletes should dress in thin layers using synthetic fabrics that promote warmth. Try to avoid overdressing. Remember what your mother said, "Wear a hat!" Nearly half of body heat is lost through the top of the head.

ALTITUDE DISORDERS

Definition

Altitude sickness and acute mountain sickness are illnesses caused by poor adjustments to the decrease in O_2 (hypoxia) encountered when exposed to a new high altitude environment. There are no specific factors that make one individual more susceptible than another. Athletes must be cautious when traveling to and competing in high altitudes at which they are not acclimatized.

Etiology

Normal O_2 concentration in the air at sea level is 21% and the barometric (air) pressure is 760 Hg. At higher altitudes, the O_2 concentration stays the same, but the barometric pressure drops and there are fewer O_2 molecules taken in per breath. In response to this environmental situation, the body will increase the respiration rate and consequently the heart rate to move the blood faster through the system, trying to meet the demands for O_2. Although the physical activity may be the same as at sea level, the body must adjust to having less O_2 to do the same task. Prolonged exposure to high altitude and lower air pressure can lead to fluid leaking from capillaries and a fluid build-up in the lungs and brain.

History and Examination

The signs of an altitude disorder usually appear when ascending to high altitudes. There can be a time lag (6 hours to 96 hours) between arrival and the onset of the symptoms. Signs and symptoms include headache, difficulty breathing and sleeping, waking early, loss of appetite, lightheadedness, fatigue, confusion, weakness, and labored breathing with exercise. Symptoms tend to be worst at night. Altitude sickness is thought to be a neurological problem caused by CNS changes.

Management and Treatment

The major cause of altitude sickness is going too high too fast. Allow time for the body to adjust to the new environment and O_2 levels. Acclimatization generally takes about 1 day to 3 days and the sickness is self-limiting. Headaches will respond to aspirin. Plan to limit the athletes' activity for a few days to allow their bodies to make the required accommodations. Athletes should stay hydrated because the act of acclimatization may lead to fluid loss. Athletes should eat a high carbohydrate diet while at high altitudes. Athletes should also avoid alcohol and other drugs, which may further depress the respiratory rate during sleep, making sleeping more difficult.

Special Considerations

More severe symptoms may occur. If the headache is more severe and does not respond to aspirin, if the athlete develops nausea and vomiting, and if muscle control and weakness are more pronounced, the individual may need more definitive care that may involve descending from the location. One quick test that can be used is to have the athlete walk in a straight line, as in a sobriety test. If the athlete fails, descent is required.

High altitude pulmonary edema (HAPE) and high altitude cerebral edema (HACE) are more dramatic forms of altitude sickness. HAPE results in fluid build-up in the lungs. HACE results in swelling of the brain. Signs and symptoms of HAPE include cyanosis, impaired mental function, tightness in the chest, extreme fatigue, and a persistent productive cough. Signs and symptoms of HACE are headache, loss or coordination and memory, hallucinations, weakness, and psychotic behavior. Advanced medical care is needed immediately in either case.

General Medical Emergencies

There are several, relatively common conditions that can create general medical emergencies that sports emergency care personnel must be prepared to address should they occur. Asthma, diabetes, and mononucleosis are conditions causing systemic problems if not treated correctly and quickly. Asthma and diabetes can both lead to death if not recognized immediately. As with the environmental disorders discussed in the previous section, prevention is the key to treatment. Pre-planning and awareness are necessary to avoid any first aid emergencies.

ASTHMA

Definition

Asthma is a chronic inflammatory lung disease that makes breathing difficult. When an attack occurs, the air passages will narrow and become congested to the point at which they function poorly, resulting in difficulty breathing.

Etiology

Asthma is a hyper-response of the bronchial passages to various stimuli. It is thought of as an allergic reaction or response to allergens or triggers in the air. Triggers include allergies, mold, dust mites, pollen, smoke, animals, cold air, exercise, and respiratory infections. Children are most affected by asthma, but the incidence of asthma diagnosis is on the rise among all ages due to increased air pollution.

History and Examination

Asthma occurs when an allergic trigger causes the air passages to react in 3 interrelated ways. First, the muscles around the bronchi will spasm or vasoconstrict. The bronchi are the tubes connecting the trachea (windpipe) with the alveoli, which are deep inside the lungs. The alveoli, or air sacks, are where O_2 and CO_2 are exchanged in the blood. The second reaction is swelling inside the bronchial passages. Finally, a build-up of mucus occurs inside the passages. These 3 changes to the bronchi make them narrower and reduce the flow of O_2 into the body and the transfer of CO_2 out of the lungs.

The most common sign of asthma is wheezing, which is a hoarse whistling sound made while exhaling. Wheezing occurs because air is trapped in the lungs. Other typical signs and symptoms of asthma are difficulty breathing, shortness of breath, tight chest, restless while sleeping, coughing, difficulty talking, and inability to catch a breath after activity. If the condition is left unchecked or proves itself difficult to treat, severe respiratory distress and respiratory arrest can occur.

Management and Treatment

Asthma can occur at any age, but the treatment undertaken is usually based on the assumption that the condition is or will become chronic. Prevention is the key to management. Avoiding known triggers and the use of medications designed to open the air passages are the 2 best ways to treat this disorder. Medication comes in 2 forms, oral and inhaled. They can be used in combination or singularly to control asthmatic attacks. Inhaled medications have fewer side effects in general, but shorter durations of action. There are 2 main types of asthma medication:

1. Quick relief or rescue medicines are designed to relieve symptoms after they start. These are known as bronchodilators. These medications open the bronchial tubes by relaxing muscle spasm in the walls of the tubes. In the event of an asthmatic attack, patients are encouraged to take puffs of the inhalers no more than 1 min to 2 min apart. Do not use more often than recommended. Too much use can cause tachycardia.

2. Control medicines are designed to prevent asthma symptoms from starting. Corticosteroids, either inhaled or oral, are examples of control medications.

It is very important for athletes to work with their doctors and learn the different medications designed to control and treat asthma. Athletic trainers and team physicians may need to re-evaluate if the condition worsens and/or the prescribed medication is not working effectively.

Special Considerations

Exercise-induced asthma (EIA) is a unique type of asthma that may be encounter by the athletic trainer. EIA is defined as bronchospasm caused by exercise. In this case physical activity is the trigger for the asthmatic symptoms. It can occur in those with known asthma or crop up in athletes that have never suffered a normal asthma attack. The cause of EIA is still not well understood. There are medications designed to control EIA that are approved by various athletic bodies, such as the International Olympic Committee. Athletic trainers and their athletes should work with their team physicians and the family physicians to ensure that proper medication is being used by the competing athlete.

Acute Breathing Difficulties

Over the last 25 years the number of asthma patients and individuals experiencing acute breathing episodes has been increasing. Sports emergency care providers may encounter the following acute breathing difficulties:

- Athletes who experience an acute breathing episode with no history of asthma. The end result of the episode may or may not have asthma as the causative factor.

- Athletes who are known asthma sufferers but who do not have their medication with them.

- Athletes who have the wind knocked out of them.

- Athletes who have breathing difficulty related to physical trauma from an injury or as a byproduct of stress or anxiety issues the athlete may be experiencing.

The signs and symptoms an individual with acute breathing difficulties may display will be similar to those of asthma such as wheezing, difficulty breathing or shortness of breath, tight chest, coughing, difficulty talking, numbness in the hands and fingers, numb lips, dry mouth, and dizziness. The athlete may start panting or hyperventilating (breathing faster than normal) and disrupt the balance of oxygen and CO_2 in the body as they try to catch their breath.

Management and Treatment

First try to calm and reassure the athlete. Get the athlete in a comfortable position or a better posture position. Move him or her into a fresh air location. Work with the athlete to control his or her breathing rate and pattern. Have the athlete focus on following you as you demonstrate taking long slow breaths in through the nose and long exhalations out through the month. Consider having the athlete breath into his or her cupped hands. What you are trying to accomplish is having the athlete gain voluntary control of his or her breathing. If an athlete is a known asthma sufferer, try and get some of his or her medication from his or her locker, dorm, or parents.

It is of utmost importance to try and keep minor, nonemergency breathing difficulties from becoming major problems. Sports emergency care providers should continually monitor the athlete, access his or her breathing rate, skin color, alertness, and mental function. Use a stethoscope to listen to the chest and the athlete's lung sounds. If the athlete's condition does not improve quickly or becomes serious, the health care provider should access 9-1-1 for EMS assistance and transport. Follow up care is necessary to identify the cause. Again, it is very important for athletes, their parents, primary physicians, specialists, and the sports medicine team to work together to control and treat asthma and all breathing disorders.

DIABETES

Definition

Diabetes mellitus is a disorder of carbohydrate metabolism resulting from inadequate production or utilization of insulin and inefficient use of blood sugar.

Etiology

Insulin is a hormone secreted by the pancreas. It is essential in the metabolism of glucose (simple sugar). It helps promote the storage of glucose in muscles and in the liver in the form of glycogen. Insulin also helps control the transfer of glucose from the blood into skeletal and cardiac muscles. To function normally, the body cells need a proper balance of sugar and insulin. Diabetes can seriously affect the body in a variety of ways and contribute to other conditions such as blindness; kidney, heart, and tooth disease; and strokes.

History and Examination

Athletes with diabetes can compete if they are able to maintain blood sugar levels within normal limits. If the condition is not controlled properly, the

athlete will have too much or too little sugar in the bloodstream. This imbal
ance will lead to a diabetic emergency.

There are 2 types of diabetes. In Type I, or insulin-dependent diabetes,
the pancreas produces little or no insulin. This type of individual will need
to monitor his blood sugar regularly and inject insulin several times per day.
Type I diabetes is also called juvenile diabetes. In Type II diabetes (non–insulin-dependent diabetes), the body produces insulin, but either not enough or
the cells do not use the insulin effectively. Type II is also called adult-onset
diabetes and is much more common than Type I. Most people with Type II are
able to regulate their blood sugar through diet and oral medication. There are
2 types of diabetic emergencies. When the level of insulin in the body is too
low, the blood sugar levels will be too high and the athlete will suffer from
hyperglycemia. In this condition, although there is enough glucose in the
blood, it cannot be transported from the bloodstream. The cells in the body,
needing food or glucose, will try to get energy from other stored foods, such
as fats. Turning fat into energy is not efficient and will create a lot of waste
products in the blood and the athlete will become ill. This is called diabetic
ketoacidosis. Signs and symptoms of diabetic ketoacidosis are hot, dry skin
and a sweet, fruity breath odor. This can be mistaken for alcohol on the
breath. A life-threatening condition known as diabetic coma may occur if
diabetic ketoacidosis is not treated properly.

In hypoglycemia, the level of insulin in the body is too high and the glucose
levels in the blood will be too low. Sugar is used up too fast. Left untreated, the
athlete will develop insulin shock, another life-threatening condition.

Hypoglycemia and hyperglycemia have different causes and different
symptoms (Table 12-9).

Management and Treatment

Diabetes is not a reason for an individual to stop participating in athletics.
In fact, exercise can help to control diabetes and increase insulin efficiency.
However, the athlete needs to understand the necessary balance between diet
and exercise. Regular monitoring of the blood sugar should be done with a
glucose monitor.

Insulin injections may become a thing of the past in the future as researchers look for and test new delivery methods. One promising delivery method
that has already gained widespread acceptance, especially for athletes, is the
insulin pump. The pump mimics the normal regular release of insulin from
the pancreas. The pump is not automatic; the user decides how much insulin
will be given. These pumps weigh about 3 oz and are about the size of a cell
phone and worn like a beeper on the belt or in the pocket. These units are
computerized and programmed to give regular insulin 24 hours a day. The
pumps have a small flexible catheter tube with a fine needle on the end, which
is inserted under the skin of the abdomen. The needle is normally taped in

Table 12-9

SIGNS AND SYMPTOMS OF HYPOGLYCEMIA AND HYPERGLYCEMIA

Hypoglycemia	Hyperglycemia
Sudden onset	Gradual onset
Pale, cool, clammy skin	Flushed, warm, dry skin
Mood changes, disorientation, confusion, or stupor	Frequent urination
Unresponsiveness (late stages)	Fruity or sweet odor on breath
	Irregular breathing
	Drowsiness, disorientation, or stupor
	Nausea, feeling and looking ill
	Unresponsiveness (late stages)

place. Frequent monitoring is still necessary to maintain the proper glucose and insulin balance. Specially designed and padded waist belts are available for use in athletic competition.

To treat an athlete experiencing a diabetic emergency, check for life-threatening conditions. If the athlete's past medical history is unknown, look for a medic alert tag or ask bystanders if they know if the athlete has diabetes. Most diabetic emergencies are hypoglycemic in nature. If the athlete is conscious, give him or her some form of sugar. Commercially available glucose paste is available for use and should be kept in every medical kit. Other alternatives such as cake icing or table sugar, candy, fruit juice, or soda will contain enough sugar to help restore a normal balance; however, do not give a victim food or drink if he or she is experiencing an altered state of consciousness. Glucose paste, cake icing, and sugar can be placed under the tongue. If it is unclear whether the diabetic emergency is due to hypoglycemia or hyperglycemia, give sugar. If the sugar levels are low, recovery will be rapid. If they are too high, the additional sugar will not harm the athlete.

Prevention is again a key with athletes. Taking the time to review the condition with diabetic athletes and their coaches may be very helpful. Items to consider include the following:

- Be sure the condition is properly documented on the preseason physical form and review the condition with the athlete so you are aware of his or her normal management plan.

- The diabetes should be well controlled before practice starts.
- Practices and games should be held at the same basic time of day and be about the same length.
- Have sugary snacks on hand to help balance out irregularities.
- Since the legs and arms will be used in activity, only give insulin injections in the abdomen.
- Be sure to maintain proper hydration. Remember fluid is vitally important for all bodily functions.
- Be ready to test the athlete's blood glucose before and regularly during exercise.
- Regularly review the exercise plan and make adjustments.

Usually, most diabetics will be familiar with their condition and know how best to treat it. Ask for their help. If the individual is not feeling better after 5 minutes, call 9-1-1. Obviously, if he or she is unconscious, call 9-1-1 immediately, and do not give anything orally. Monitor and document vital signs until EMS arrives.

MONONUCLEOSIS

Definition

Mononucleosis is a common infectious disease that can affect the liver, lymph nodes, and oral cavity.

Etiology

Mononucleosis is usually caused by the Epstein-Barr virus (EBV), a member of the herpes family of viruses. It gets its name from the traumatic increase in the number of white blood cells (mononuclear leukocytes) that are created when the EBV infects the lymphatic system in the body. The lymphatic system is the complex disease-fighting system in the body and is made up of the following parts: bone marrow, spleen, thymus gland, lymph nodes, tonsils, and appendix.

The disease is mostly seen in adolescents and young adults aged 15 to 30 but can occur at any age. The disease is contracted through direct contact with saliva or mucus of an infected individual and is commonly transmitted by sharing food or drink containers or by kissing, giving it its description as the "kissing disease." Some newly infected athletes may not have symptoms and may potentially spread the virus to others.

History and Examination

The incubation time for this disease is usually 2 weeks to 7 weeks. The symptoms will last a few days to a couple of months, most often disappearing in 1 week to 3 weeks. The signs and symptoms are rather vague and start with the athlete having a general fatigue or run-down feeling. This feeling may come and go. The person will feel he or she has a bad cold or the flu. Common additional symptoms include headache, chills, loss of appetite, and puffy eyes. As the athlete typically tries to fight through the disease, the symptoms will worsen and he or she will experience swollen, tender glands, high fever, sore throat, and fatigue. The athlete will want to sleep often because he or she will never feel fully rested. As stated previously, the white blood cell count will be elevated and lymphatic system will be on full alert, with the spleen enlarged.

Athletes with these symptoms need to be referred to a medical professional for testing. An antibody blood test, "monospot," will be done to confirm the diagnosis and eliminate other possibilities.

Management and Treatment

There is no specific treatment for this disease. Basic treatment will be rest, taking acetaminophen or ibuprofen, and eating and drinking properly. This usually mild disease will run its course in a few weeks. Again, the symptoms may come and go. The sore throat will be worst during days 3 to 5, gradually improving by day 10. The fever may last 2 weeks. The athlete once diagnosed should stay away from practice and school until the fever goes away and he or she feels more rested. The athlete will be encouraged not to push it or try to rush the process. The glands may stay swollen for almost 1 month.

Special Considerations

Sports emergency care personnel must be concerned about athletes with mononucleosis because of the enlarged spleen and the increased chance of rupturing it during activity. A splenic rupture is a medical emergency and can be life threatening. Contact sports and heavy lifting should be avoided. Return-to-play considerations must be made after an ultrasound test is done to ensure the spleen has returned to normal size and the white blood cell count has returned to somewhat normal levels.

Reference

1. Thomas CL, ed. *Taber's Cyclopedic Medical Dictionary*. 19th ed. Philadelphia: FA Davis; 1997.

Bibliography

American Diabetes Association. About insulin pumps. Available at: http://www.diabetes.org/for-parents-for-kids/diabetes-care/insulin-pumps.jsp. Accessed November 23, 2006.

American Red Cross. *Emergency Response*. Yardley, Pa: Staywell; 2001.

American Red Cross. *Professional Rescuer CPR*. Yardley, Pa: Staywell; 2006.

American Red Cross. *Responding to Emergency.* Yardley, Pa. Staywell, 2000.

Binkley H, Beckett J, Casa D, Kleiner D, Plummer P. NATA position statement: exertional heat illness. *Journal of Athletic Training.* 2002;37(3):329-343.

Cerny F, Burton H. *Exercise Physiology for Health Care Professionals.* Champaign, Ill: Human Kinetics Publishers; 2001.

Curtis R. Outdoor action guide to high altitude: acclimatization and illness. Available at: http://www.princeton.edu/~oa/safety/altitude.html. Accessed November 12, 2006.

Food and Drug Administration. On the teen scene: being a sport with exercise-induced asthma. Available at: http://www.fda.gov/fdac/reprints/ots_asth.html. Accessed November 14, 2006.

Institute of Medicine of the National Academies. Dietary reference intakes: water, potassium, sodium, chloride, and sulfate. Available at: http://wwwion.edu/?id=18495andredirect=0. Accessed November 23, 2006.

Magee D. *Orthopedic Physical Assessment.* 2nd ed. Philadelphia: WB Saunders Company; 1992.

McArdle W, Katch F, Katch V. *Sports and Exercise Nutrition.* Baltimore, Md: Lippincott Williams and Wilkins; 1999.

Miller M, Weiler J, Baker R, Collins J, D'Alonzo G. NATA position statement: management of asthma in athletes. *Journal of Athletic Training.* 2005;40(3):224-245.

National Athletic Trainers Association. Inter-Association task force on exertional heat illness consensus statement. 2003. Availablet at: http://www.nata.org/statements/consensus/heatillness.pdf. Accessed March 29, 2007.

National Safety Council. *First Aid and CPR.* 4th ed. Sudbury, Mass: Jones and Bartlett Publishers; 2000.

National Weather Service. Heat wave: a major summer killer. Available at: http://www.nws.noaa.gov/om/brochures/heat_wave.shtml. Accessed November 12, 2006.

Papazian R. On the teen scene: being a sport with exercise-induced asthma. Available at: http://www.gssiweb.com. Accessed November 3, 2006.

Perrin D, ed. *Assessment of Athletic Injuries.* Champaign, Ill: Human Kinetics Publishers; 2000.

Starkey C. *Athletic Training and Sports Medicine.* 4th ed. Sudbury, Mass: Jones & Bartlett Publishers; 2006.

Starkey C, Ryan J. *Evaluation of Orthopedic and Athletic Injuries.* 2nd ed. Philadelphia: FA Davis; 2002.

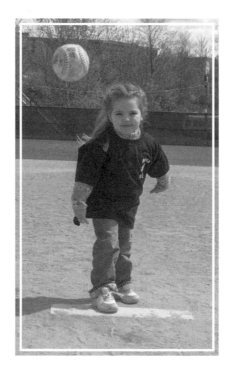

Emergency Care Considerations for the Pediatric and Youth Athlete

Chapter 13

Jeff G. Konin, PhD, ATC, PT

There has been a significant increase in the number of youths participating in organized and recreational sports over the past decade.[1] In particular, a dramatic rise has been seen in the number of youths participating in such sports as softball, Pop Warner Football, and soccer. As such, both the overall number of injuries and the severity of these injuries have grown in volume.[2,3] The increases in participation and injury rates have been attributed to a number of factors, including but not limited to, the federal government's passing of Title IX legislation allowing for greater equality for female athletic participation; a recent level of interest for certain youth sports such as soccer; increased media coverage of sports such as gymnastics, skating, tennis, and swimming; and a greater-than-ever emphasis on competition driven by year-round desires to improve skill and conditioning levels for hopes of obtaining collegiate-level scholarships to offset the cost of a college education.[3] According to recent data reported by the National Athletic Trainers' Association (NATA), the National SAFE CHILDREN Campaign, and the American Academy of Pediatrics (AAP), approximately 775,000 children aged 15 and under have sought emergency medical care for a sports-related injury, many the potential result of parents being unsure of how to determine the seriousness of an injury or illness.[4-6] Furthermore, children ages 5 to 14 account for nearly 40% of all sports-related injuries treated in hospital emergency departments.[5] Boys ages 10 to 14 are twice as likely as girls of the same age to be treated in a hospital emergency room for a sports-related injury and are also more likely than girls to suffer from multiple injuries simultaneously.

Professional medical care is absent at the majority of organized youth sporting activities. With few exceptions, such as national tournament-like events (ie, Little League World Series), emergency medical care is managed impromptu, without any advanced planning, and by a coach or parent who is most comfortable aiding and assisting an injured individual, though this person may not be medically credentialed or qualified in any such manner to provide formal care. While the "Good Samaritan" approach is appreciated, it does not reflect the optimal standard of care. More importantly, it could potentially lead to more harmful and/or mishandled circumstances.[7,8] Outside of organized sporting events for today's youth, the involvement with higher risk activities via the use of trampolines, in-lines skates, and other activities has also spawned an increase in traumatic injuries to children, oftentimes without any parental supervision, leading to nontreatment or a delay in the treatment of medical emergencies.

One should not be too naïve to recognize that providing on-site professional medical care at all youth sporting events regardless of the level of competition is solely an issue of cost. However, this fact should not mislead the public into realizing that the risk and severity of injuries sustained by children is of less importance than to those sustained by adults. In fact, in many cases, the risk, prevalence, and severity are of greater concern given the immaturity of a child's anatomical features and underdevelopment of certain vital organs. Given the predicted continual growth identified with youth sport involvement, it would behoove parents and others to adapt improved guidelines for emergency care of traumatic-type injuries to children.

Prevention of Youth Sport Emergencies

Much debate exists within the medical community as to whether or not injuries can actually be prevented, let alone acute traumatic and unpredictable types of injuries. Despite the lack of evidence, the majority of medical professionals believe that there are some common sense prevention measures that can be taken in an effort to identify potential risk factors for injury and illness among children participating in sports.

PREPARTICIPATION PHYSICAL EXAMINATIONS

Several professional associations have teamed together to identify the PPPE as the gold standard for assessment (Table 13-1).[9] The purpose of the PPPE is to provide for a more sports-specific assessment of an individual, not to replace the standard physical examination performed by a physician during a typical and routine office visit. Depending upon the approach, a single physician can perform such an assessment or a multitude of individuals can collaborate in a team-like manner and perform a station-based PPPE. Lombardo first described the PPPE in 1994, identifying the following reasons for performing a PPPE, and later others endorsed a similar evidence-based approach to the PPPE[10-12]:

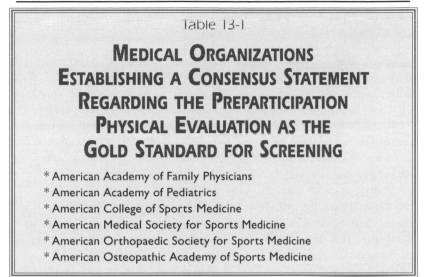

Table 13-1

MEDICAL ORGANIZATIONS ESTABLISHING A CONSENSUS STATEMENT REGARDING THE PREPARTICIPATION PHYSICAL EVALUATION AS THE GOLD STANDARD FOR SCREENING

* American Academy of Family Physicians
* American Academy of Pediatrics
* American College of Sports Medicine
* American Medical Society for Sports Medicine
* American Orthopaedic Society for Sports Medicine
* American Osteopathic Academy of Sports Medicine

Table 13-2

RECOMMENDED PORTIONS OF A STANDARDIZED EXAMINATION

* Medical history questionnaire	* Weight and height
* General appearance	* Blood pressure
* Vision	* Cardiovascular
* Respiratory	* Neurological
* Abdominal/genitourinary	* Musculoskeletal
* Integumentary	

- To gather baseline data for future reference
- To detect manageable medical conditions that may interfere with sports participation
- To determine whether there are contraindications to participation
- To serve as a limited general health screening
- To fulfill legal requirements

Table 13-2 identifies components recommended as portions of a standardized examination.[13-15]

It is suggested that an examination be performed within 6 weeks of the beginning of participation. This would allow for both recent medical conditions to be identified and present with ample time to perform any further medical and/or laboratory tests with definitive results and findings prior to the start of one's participation time frame.[14]

In today's world, some form of PPPE appears to be the standard acceptance of clearance prior to formal organized participation. However, some in the medical profession question whether or not certain aspects of the examination are worth performing since they yield such low prevalence rates of findings. Numerous musculoskeletal findings that would be classified as "deficits" or perhaps "non-normative" have not been demonstrated to be the causative factor of any eventual catastrophic or even mild injury. Magnes et al reported on 10,540 pre-season evaluations on children between the ages of 10 to 19 over a 5-year period and found that overall 47 (0.4%) failed the exam, 18 (0.2%) had hypertension, 6 (0.06%) presented with blindness, 5 (0.06%) were absent a testicle, and 4 (0.05%) had postconcussion symptoms.[16] With such small numbers of conditions being identified, the resources of time and money are questioned as to their worth in performing such lengthy exams.

Best feels as though the PPPE has minimal effect on overall mortality and morbidity associated with sport participation and that no standard PPPE exists whereby a true consensus is found.[17] Furthermore, Best states that there is no clear consensus on who should perform the PPPE, and that in fact a proper medical history may be more effective than the clinical exam itself.[17]

Briskin et al in 2006 concluded that among highly active female adolescent dancers, a history of compromised bone quality was significantly associated with a predictive finding of a stress fracture. This finding is suggestive of dual emission x-ray absorptiometry (DXA) scanning when working with this population as a means of being proactive when the recognition of lower bone mineral density is present.[18] A proactive approach may prevent more significant and complicated acute fractures that take longer to heal and may ultimately impact long-term athletic activity.

Some sudden death conditions resulting from athletic participation appear to be undetectable during a PPPE. For example, according to Maron et al[19]:

- 1 in 10 sudden deaths in young people are associated with sports.
- One hundred fifty-eight deaths occurred between 1985 to 1995, of which 24 (15%) were attributable to noncardiovascular causes.
- Of the 134 remaining, 120 deaths were in males and due to a variety of causes of which the most common was hypertrophic cardiomyopathy.
- One hundred fifteen of the 158 had a PPPE, but only 4 were suspected of having cardiovascular disease and in only one was the lesion identified correctly.

The American Academy of Pediatrics has identified certain medical conditions that can be used to determine if participation would create an increased risk of injury or adversely affect the medical condition itself.[6] While the list

Table 13-3

MEDICAL CONDITIONS REQUIRING POTENTIAL FURTHER INQUIRY PRIOR TO ALLOWING SPORTS PARTICIPATION

* Atlantoaxial injury
* Bleeding disorders
* Cardiovascular disease
* Congenital heart disease
* Hypertension
* Dysrhythmia
* Heart murmur
* Cerebral palsy
* Diabetes mellitus
* Diarrhea
* Eating disorders (anorexia nervosa, bulimia)
* Visual deficits (loss of an eye, detached retina)
* Fever
* Heat illness
* Hepatitis
* Human immunodeficiency virus infection
* Kidney disease
* Liver disease
* Malignant neoplasm
* Musculoskeletal disorders
* Neurologic disorders (concussion, epilepsy)
* Obesity
* Organ transplant recipient
* Ovary (absence of one)
* Respiratory conditions (asthma, upper respiratory infection)
* Sickle cell disease
* Skin disorders (boils, herpes simplex, impetigo, scabies, *molluscum contagiosum*)
* Spleen enlargement
* Testicle (undescending or absence of one)

may not be all-inclusive since circumstances vary, this type of information is found to be valuable during a PPPE when one needs to determine the status of sports participation eligibility (Table 13-3). These decisions are oftentimes not

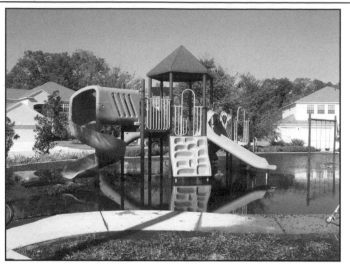

Figure 13-1. A neighborhood playground with puddles that could lead to children slipping and getting hurt.

black and white, and in fact may be quite complex and challenging. An exam should not only include written criteria that are identified as suggested guidelines, but also clinical expertise of the physician, recommendations of other expert physicians, the current health status of the athlete, the specific sport, the athlete's position, and its inherent risks, among other considerations.

Field Safety

Unfortunately, many injuries that are preventable are the result of poor field conditions. Traumatic injuries can be the result of carelessness in maintaining a safe playing environment. In general, field safety is an area of prevention that can be practiced by all parties involved with youth sports, including parents, coaches, and community recreational employees. A systematic approach should be taken and documented on a regular basis to assess the safety status of all playing surfaces and equipment. Some of the items to be considered as possibly leading to a higher incidence of injury risk include the following:

- Uneven playing surfaces
- Surfaces with greater than normal friction (ie, old hardwood courts)
- Slippery playing surfaces (ie, fields with puddles) (Figure 13-1)
- Improper lighting for night events
- Irrigation systems not completely buried (Figure 13-2)
- Baseball dugouts without proper protection from hit balls

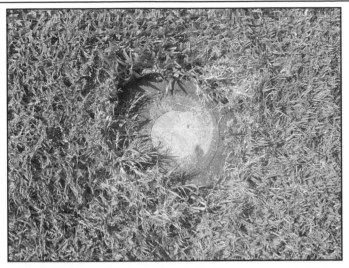

Figure 13-2. An example of a sprinkler head at a ball field that is not properly maintained for safety precautions.

- Fences that surround fields with protruding parts
- Goalposts and other fixed apparatus that are not properly protected with padding

Equipment Safety

All equipment that is used, and especially that reissued on an annual basis as part of a recreational or organized program, should be carefully inspected and repaired as needed and according to any standards or guidelines that may exist. This may include baseball bats, gloves, pads, braces, and masks. Protective equipment serves numerous functions according to Konin and McCue and therefore should be kept in current functioning order.[20] These functions include, but are not limited to, absorbing forces, limiting anatomical movements, supporting joint structures and musculotendinous structures, enhancing proprioceptive feedback, and securing protective pads.[20] In general, any equipment issued or reissued should be properly fitted and sized, specifically helmets for sports such as football and ice hockey and shoulder pads for football, ice hockey, and lacrosse.[15] Loose-fitting helmets and shoulder pads can lead to a greater impact of forces sustained through direct contact, potentially leading to more serious injuries. In particular as it relates to younger children and those playing a sport for the first time, feedback regarding poor-fitting braces, pads, or helmets may not be accurate (Figure 13-3). Thus, individuals with knowledge should be involved with appropriate equipment issuing.

Figure 13-3. Example of an improperly fitted facemask for baseball that is too big for the size of the child.

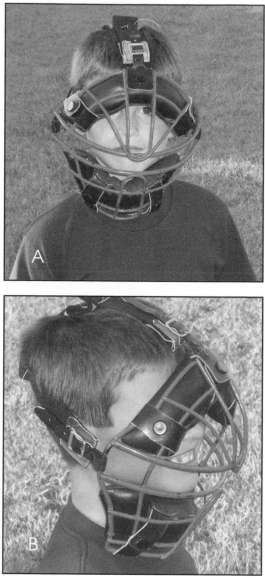

Recently, some sports/events have placed an emphasis on certain pieces of protective equipment as both a response from adverse experiences and/or data demonstrating a high incidence of specific injuries. These include pole vault, women's lacrosse, field hockey, football, men's lacrosse, baseball, soccer, and mouth guards.

POLE VAULT

As a result of the potential risk associated with awkward and unprepared landings, even some possibly beyond the limits of the protective matted landing cushion, helmets have now been designed specifically for vaulters. These helmets are composed of a carbon and e-glass composite shell and weigh about as much or less than a standard bicycle helmet. In addition, the vault box is now made with a "soft box" soft cushion inner lining to further pad the athlete's landing.

WOMEN'S LACROSSE

Effective January 1, 2005, the sport of women's lacrosse at the intercollegiate level mandated the use of protective eyewear. This was the result of a rash of eye and facial injuries, and thus established the goal of prevention of rare but catastrophic eye injuries. The American Society for Testing and Materials (ASTM) approves such eyewear and believes that the eye protection used should be able to withstand forces of 45 miles per hour (mph) for youth and 60 mph for adults. Lacrosse associations within the United States have been proactive in educating youth athletes on how to obtain eyewear that has been proven and tested to sustain such forces.

FIELD HOCKEY

Recently, collaboration has occurred between the NCAA Field Hockey Committee and equipment manufacturers to develop eyewear that will promote extended views while providing for optimal protection. As products are developed from research and collaboration at the professional and intercollegiate levels, these same pieces of equipment will be designed for children to afford them the same level of safety as their adult counterparts.

FOOTBALL

Tinted face shields have become a trend for many athletes in the sport of football. However, complaints have been leveled against these nontransparent, or nonclear, shields because it is difficult to see another player's eyes behind them. This posed concerns for both medical personnel as well as football players themselves when playing against one another. As a result, the NCAA has established guidelines for the use of a nontransparent eye shield that now include the following steps for an exemption to wear such a shield[15]:

- Completed request form from rules committees.
- Request made on university/medical professional letterhead with appropriate signatures.
- NCAA Committee on Competitive Safeguards and Medical Aspects of Sport will review requests.
- Written notification will be provided.
- Approvals are made per annum.
- Appeals may be reviewed with additional information.

The American Academy of Pediatrics in 2004 issued advice pertaining to protective eyewear for young athletes. A summary of the bullet points includes the following[6]:

- All children are encouraged to wear appropriate eye protection if participating in a sport that poses a risk of eye injury.
- Proper fit is essential.
- Three-mm polycarbonate lenses should be used for children with narrow faces who cannot fit well in goggles.
- Goggles approved by the American National Standards Institute (ANSI) are considered to be of the gold standard.
- Wearing contact lenses offers no protection in and of itself.
- Functional athletes with one eye should wear protection.

The Protective Eyewear Certification Council (PECC) also exists to test for standards in eyewear. Eyewear approved in the laboratory for adults is considered acceptable for youth as well. Currently, no guidelines exist for eyeglass wearers, and goggles are not designed to cover standard eyeglasses.[21] With respect to actual competitions, game officials only assess that eyewear is worn; they do not have the capability to assess if appropriate standard eyewear protection is being used. Parents, coaches, and medical providers must take the responsibility to assure that appropriate protection is being implemented. The recent findings of reported orofacial injuries seen in children's sports will continue to place this issue at the forefront of those involved with caring for such traumatic incidents.[22,23]

MEN'S LACROSSE

Men's lacrosse, though contact in nature, has gone relatively unscathed with respect to catastrophic injuries until late. As a result of a rash of deaths related to commotio cordis, 4 of which involved men's lacrosse players over the past 5 years, a summit discussing the condition was formed that included representatives from United States Lacrosse, the NATA, the NCAA, the

American College of Sports Medicine, The American Medical Society for Sports Medicine, and youth baseball equipment manufacturers.[24-28] To date, discussion has surrounded the weight (5 oz) and material (rubber) of the ball, the speed at which the ball travels (up to 90 mph), and the time frame whereby blunt trauma to the heart can lead to ventricular fibrillation (20 mSec window). An emphasis on research in this area has been established and the use of good preparation that includes effective emergency action plans with an on-site AED is now considered the standard of care for this arena.

BASEBALL

The sport of baseball is also entertaining discussion regarding catastrophic injuries that could potentially occur. Though rare, commotio cordis is also a concern, especially to the individual playing the catcher position. At ball speeds of 40 mph, the risk of commotio cordis is greatest, and when the speeds increase, the risk decreases. However, the 40 mph speed is closely related to the speeds seen with Little League throwers. Recommendations have been made to include using baseballs with softer core insides as well as using thermoplast-molded chest protectors.[29] This concern as it relates to baseball has not yet received the same level of attention as it has with lacrosse.

SOCCER

The sport of soccer has not experienced a wave of catastrophic injuries despite its growing popularity throughout the world. However, it has not gone without some discussion regarding ways to reduce the number of serious head injuries experienced when colliding with the goal posts as well as from player-to-player direct contact. Questions have been raised as to whether or not goal posts should be changed from wood and metal to vinyl or padded. Currently, the main issue appears to be related to safety versus cost. That is, are there enough catastrophic head injuries that warrant a mandate that will cost millions of dollars to change the equipment? Published reports of Injury Surveillance Systems (ISS) show very low incidence of the need to justify such a change at this time.[15]

MOUTH GUARDS

Protective mouth guards are an important piece of equipment for anyone exposed to the risk of contact or collision to the facial area (Figure 13-4).[15] This includes not only sports such as football and wrestling, but sports such as basketball and soccer in which someone's elbow may accidentally hit another player in the mouth, and sports like ice hockey, field hockey, and lacrosse where a ball traveling at high speeds can hit a player in the mouth. Various forms of mouth guards exist, ranging from the standard shelf-stocked to the

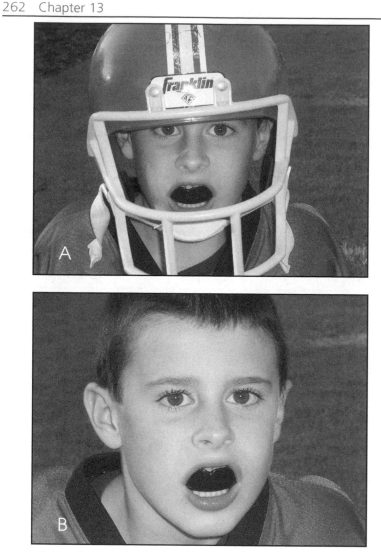

Figure 13-4. An example of a mouth guard used for youth sports.

custom fitted and formed types. As one would expect, more protection is afforded with the mouth guards that are custom formed.

Sporting Rules

While some catastrophic and acute emergency-like injuries are not preventable and are unfortunately accepted as part of the sport in which one participates, others can be prevented through rule changes. Of greatest note is in the sport of football, where the rules related to how one tackles, specifically the avoidance of "spearing," have been implemented at all levels of play.[15]

In all sports, league officials and referees have taken a stronger stance against flagrant play and unsportsmanlike conduct in an effort to prevent unnecessary severe injuries. This vigilance against such play not only prevents immediate injury, but potentially long-term complications and recurrent inappropriate behavior.

Little league baseball has implemented rules that relate to limiting the number of pitches a child can throw in any given day and/or week. This is not likely designed to prevent an acute emergency, but rather long-term damage to one's upper extremity at a young age that can develop through chronic overuse.[30] Though the rules have good intentions, honest enforcement and the fact that many children nowadays actually play in multiple leagues simultaneously with no method of monitoring the number of overall throws in a given time frame pose difficulty in actual quantitative interventions. At this time, no episodes of acute emergencies such as fractures or dislocations related to excessive throwing in a child have been reported.

Physical and Psychological Immaturity

Medical emergencies can occur to children in slightly different ways than they do with adults for a variety of reasons. Children's bodies are still growing and their coordination is still developing and therefore, their physical and emotional maturity levels are not on par with those of an adult. Prior to puberty, girls and boys are likely to experience the same risk of sports injuries. However, during puberty, boys will experience a greater number of injuries and more severe injuries than girls. The American Academy of Pediatrics recommends that late-developing teens avoid contact sports until their bodies have developmentally "caught up" to their peer's body sizes because children and adolescents who are less developed than a more mature child or adolescent of the same age and weight are at increased risk of injury.[6]

In general, young children may not be able to accurately assess the risks associated with participating in certain sports. They are lacking in various aspects of physical maturity, such as having slightly less developed coordination skills, slower reaction times, and less accuracy as it relates to movement patterns. Imbalances in muscular development can lead to muscle strains and avulsion-type fractures. As such, sports that involve greater levels of contact, collision, or even sudden, rapid movements tend to pose a greater risk of injury. Those who are just beginning to partake in a sport for the first time are also more susceptible to acquiring an injury, especially one of greater magnitude as a result of the lack of knowledge and awareness of the sport.

Anatomically, a child is at greater risk of physical injury merely due to the fact that aspects of his or her musculoskeletal system are not yet fully developed. Children who sustain fractures that involve immature growth plates will need to be assessed carefully to determine the extent of the injury. In some cases, such fractures can be treated very conservatively, and healing will occur rather quickly without a high percentage of potential complications. On the other hand, if a significant disruption occurs to an immature growth plate, more aggressive intervention may be needed to secure adequate circulation in an attempt to prevent premature closure. It is important to identify such situations as early as possible so as to not compromise any potential outcome.[31-34]

Thoracic wall injuries are commonplace among pediatric and adolescent children. In fact, Sartorelli and Vane identify thoracic trauma as the second leading cause of death in children, behind brain injuries.[35] Although these types of injuries are not seen as often in children as they are in adults, they remain a source of morbidity and mortality.[36] The compliant chest wall of children affords far more opportunistic injuries such as pulmonary contusions and rib fractures.[35] In addition, children's thoracic wall anatomy and physiology differ from that of an adult with respect to pulmonary function, residual capacity, blood volume, chest wall and spinal soft tissue mobility, and cardiac function.[36] Neve et al have shown that both lung and thoracic development occur during and until the end of puberty in the adolescent male. Conversely, in adolescent females, lung development is almost finished following menarche.[37]

Traumatic abdominal wall herniations (TAWH) have been described in the literature more commonly as of late, with an emphasis on the etiology coming from a bicycle accident and the subsequent force of the abdominal wall hitting the handlebars (Figure 13-5).[38-44] Children as young as 7 years old have suffered intra-abdominal injuries, while in many cases surgical intervention was required.[40,43] Similar types of injuries have also been reported in children under the age of 17 taking part in alpine skiing activities, particularly trauma to the kidneys.[45] Storsved et al described a case of a congenital solitary kidney (renal agenesis) in a 17-year-old offensive lineman who landed on his backside while participating in the sport of football. The youth presented with typical findings such as pain in the lower back and gluteal region, radiating pain down the leg, and shortness of breath. A CAT scan revealed a hematoma without renal abnormality and the absence of a right kidney. Renal agenesis is very rare, and no evidence exists regarding the risk of return to a sport, particularly one such as football.[46]

Identifying physical injuries in a child, especially those of an emergent nature, can oftentimes be a challenge because children do not always possess the psychological maturity to accurately convey their perceived levels of pain and discomfort. It is not uncommon for a child to actually sustain a fracture and complain of pain, but the parent or coach writes it off as anything

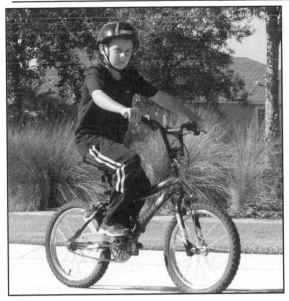

Figure 13-5. The position of the handlebars on a child's bike are such that any sudden stop of the bike would propel a child forward with the handlebars pushing up against the chest and abdominal wall area.

from a simple "bruise" to a "growing pain." The same child only hours later may even be playing actively in the backyard with a fractured arm or leg. It is only several days later that the fracture is identified. Furthermore, referral patterns from injuries to internal organs may not be identified or accurately reported by a child. Another area of recent concern is symptoms reported by a child following a concussion and how accurate the subjective history may be. A head injury sustained by a child may in fact be more severe than that suffered by an adult due to the ongoing neurocognitive development of the child's brain.[47,48] This is an area of research that is in its infancy. One interesting finding that has been reported by Broshek et al is that following a sustained concussion, female athletes tend to have significantly greater declines in both simple and complex reaction times when compared to baseline testing prior to the concussion.[49] This same work found that females report more symptoms postconcussion than males of similar circumstances. In fact, females were found to be nearly 1.7 times more cognitively impaired versus males following a concussion. One should keep this in mind and not always consider such reporting of a greater number of symptoms as a magnified result related to a more severe injury.

It is important to mention that along with the physical immaturity associated with identifying children's injuries, there is also psychological immaturity as well. Part of this rests on the shoulders of a child who has not yet formulated adult-like thought processes, and yet another part of the blame falls on overzealous parents. Moreso than ever before, parents will put added pressures on their children to not only participate, but in fact to succeed in sports at high levels. Children participate in recreational teams, travel teams, and other organized forms of competition year round, and sometimes more than one team simultaneously. This has led to an abundance of overuse injuries from the physiological perspective, but also feelings of burnout, disinterest, and even withdrawal from a child who is being pushed to play without an adequate level of self-enjoyment. Participation as the result of external pressures can lead to a child not paying attention to detail and ultimately can be the cause of a potentially dangerous situation, resulting in a severe injury.

Emergency Action Plans

Injuries of an emergency type are unavoidable; they will occur due to the very nature of athletic and activity participation. From anaphylactic reactions as the result of a bee sting to being hit in the head with a pitched ball, it is critical to have a plan in place to manage such concerning situations. An EAP, though standardized in nature, must be developed by vested individuals and relate specifically to a venue and its geographical surroundings.

EAPs should be developed, reviewed, and revised by individuals familiar with the venues of play, administrators, medical personnel, coaches, parents, legal counsel, and others who have keen awareness to detail. Table 13-4 includes a list of items to consider when drafting such a plan. The EAP should be rehearsed on a scheduled basis and at all times when new personnel, coaching staff, or others are involved with leadership roles. Components of the plan should also involve a minimal skill set expectation, with coaches and league officials being certified in CPR and the use of AED at a minimum. Written copies of the plan should be disseminated to anyone involved with expectations of intervening in an emergency situation, and the plan should be posted in plain sight and in legible format for those present to identify with in the case of an emergency.

Lastly, parents and coaches should possess additional awareness of how to respond to emergencies involving children with a higher risk of injury. For example, if a child playing youth soccer is diabetic, then coaches of that team should have such knowledge of this condition and at the bare minimum know how to recognize warning signs of a diabetic coma or insulin shock, as well as know how to initially react in such cases. As previously discussed, a good prevention plan can have a tremendous impact on properly managing emergency situations.

Today, all professional and college/university sports medicine programs have documented and implemented various forms of an EAP. However, the same approach for recreational, organized, and community youth sporting events lags significantly behind (Figure 13-6). Examples of well-designed

Table 13-4

COMPONENTS OF A WELL-DESIGNED EMERGENCY ACTION PLAN

* Purpose of plan (ie, goals and objectives)
* Personnel involved (ie, ATC, EMT, MD, first responders)
* Role of various personnel (ie, MD, EMT, ATC)
* Preferred methods of communication (ie, land line phone, cell phone, walkietalkie)
* Necessary equipment available (ie, AED, splints)
* Preferred methods of transportation (ie, ambulance, personal vehicle)
* Coverage plans (ie, on-site, on-call)
* Emergency contact information (ATC, EMT, MD, police)
* Procedural methods for various circumstances (ie, unforeseen evacuations)
* Geographical and textual maps and directions
* Environmental policies (ie, lightning, heat)
* Planned written collaborative procedures with local hospital (ie, helmet removal)

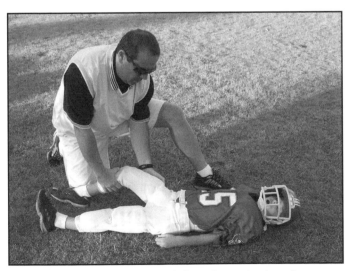

Figure 13-6. A rare, on-the-field clinical examination of an acute injury being performed on a child by a certified athletic trainer at a youth sporting event.

EAPs can be found on university sports medicine web sites and can serve as a basis of development for youth sport venue emergency action planning.[50,51]

Conclusion

Properly planned preventive measures are key to avoiding many traumatic injuries that will occur to children. PPPEs; understanding of the rules of the sport; safe, contemporary, and properly fitting equipment; and a collaborative EAP all contribute to a safe youth sport environment. The general immediate care of emergencies for pediatrics and adolescents is handled no differently than it is for adults. The appropriate first-aid assessment and required cardiopulmonary function should be assessed, stabilization of structures should occur when needed, and triage to a facility of care as soon as possible are the keys. Considerations for management of these injuries may differ once the primary vital signs are stable, so that long-term complications may be minimized or eliminated.

References

1. SNews. 2006 Participation Trends in Fitness, Sports and Outdoor Activities. Accessed from http://www.snewsnet.com/cgi-bin/snews/05751.html. Accessed on July3, 2006.

2. Methodist Hospital System. Important sports safety for the entire family. Available at: http://www.methodisthealth.com. Accessed on July 3, 2006.

3. Lindskog D. Increase in adult-type injuries among children and adolescents. Available at: http://www.ynhh.org/healthlink/pediatrics. Accessed on July 3, 2006.

4. Ingersoll CD, Sitler M, Mickalide AD, Taft AR. A national survey of parents' knowledge, attitudes and self-reported behaviors concerning sports safety. *Journal of Athletic Training*. 2001;36:S73.

5. SafeUSA. Sports injury prevention: children and adolescents. Available at: http://www.safeusa.org/sports/child.htm. Accessed on July 3, 2006.

6. American Academy of Pediatrics policy statement on medical conditions affecting sport participation. *Pediatrics*. 2001;107(5):1205-1209.

7. Allard RH. Legal aspects of sports injuries. *Ned Tijdschr Tandheelkd*. 2005;112(5):184-187.

8. Pearsall AW 4th, Kovaleski JE, Madanagopal SG. Medicolegal issues affecting sports medicine practitioners. *Clin Orthop*. 2005;(433):50-57.

9. American Academy of Family Physicians, American Academy of Pediatrics, American Medical Society of Sports Medicine, American Orthopaedic Society of Sports Medicine, and American Osteopathic Academy of Sports Medicine. *Pre-participation Physical Evaluation*. 3rd ed. Minneapolis, Minn: McGraw-Hill Companies; 2004.

10. Lombardo JA. Pre-participation physical evaluation. *Prim Care*. 1984;11(1):3-21.

Considerations for the Pediatric and Youth Athlete   269

11. Smith DM, Laskowski JA, Robinson JB. The preparticipation evaluation. *Prim Care.* 1991;18(4):777-807.
12. Lombardo JA, Badolato SK. The preparticipation physical examination. *Clin Cornerstone.* 2001;3(5):10-25.
13. Kurowski K, Chandran S. The preparticipation athletic evaluation. Available at: http://www.aafp.org/afp/20000501/2683.html. Accessed on July 3, 2006.
14. Mick TM, Dimeff RJ. What kind of physical examination does a young athlete need before participating in sports? *Cleve Clin J Med.* 2004;71(7):587-597
15. *National Collegiate Athletic Association Sports Medicine Handbook.* Indianapolis, Ind: National Collegiate Athletic Association; 2004.
16. Magnes SA, Henderson JM, Hunter SC. What conditions limit sports participation: experience with 10,540 athletes. *Phys Sports Med.* 1992;20(3):143-158.
17. Best TM. The preparticipation evaluation: an opportunity for change and consensus. *Clin J Sport Med.* 2004;14(3):107-108.
18. Briskin SM, Stanford A, Davis JH, Congeni J, Loud K. Identification of stress fracture risk factors in female college dance majors. Presented at: the 53rd Annual Meeting of the American College of Sports Medicine; Denver, Colo; June 1, 2006.
19. Maron BJ, Shirani J, Poliac LC, Mathenge R, Roberts WC, Mueller FO. Sudden death in young competitive athletes: clinical, demographic, and pathological profiles. *JAMA.* 1996;276(3):199-204.
20. Konin JG, McCue FC. Taping, bracing and strapping. In: Wilk KE, Andrews JR, eds. *The Athlete's Shoulder.* New York: Churchill Livingstone; 1994.
21. Vinger PF, Parver L, Alfaro DV, Woods T, Abrams BS. Shatter resistance of spectacle lenses. *JAMA.* 1997;277:142-144.
22. Ranalli DN, Demas PN. Orofacial injuries from sport: preventive measures for sports medicine. *Sports Med.* 2002;32(7):409-418.
23. Gordy FM, Eklund NP, DeBall S. Oral trauma in an urban emergency department. *J Dent Child (Chic).* 2004;71(1):14-116.
24. Deady B, Innes G. Sudden death of a young hockey player: case report of commotio cordis. *J Emerg Med.* 1999;17(3):459-462.
25. Kaplan JA, Karofsky PS, Volturo GA. Commotio cordis in two amateur ice hockey players despite the use of commercial chest protectors: case reports. *J Trauma.* 1993;34(1):151-153.
26. Maron BJ, Poliac JC, Kyle SS. Clinical profile of commotio cordis: an underappreciated cause of sudden cardiac death in the young during sports activities. 1997 American Heart Association Meeting. *Circulation.* 1997;96(Suppl1):1-775.
27. Maron BJ, Link MS, Wang PJ, Estes NA. Clinical profile of commotio cordis: an under appreciated cause of sudden death in the young during sports and other activities. *J Cardiovasc Electrophysiol.* 1999;10(1):114-120.
28. Link MS. Mechanically induced sudden death in chest wall impact (commotio cordis. *Prog Biophys Mol Biol.* 2003;82(1-3):175-186.

29. Weinstock J, Maron BJ, Song C, Mane PP, Estes NA, Link MS. Failure of commercially available chest wall protectors to prevent sudden cardiac death induced by chest wall blows in an experimental model of commotio cordis. *Pediatrics.* 2006;117(4):656-672.

30. Salvo JP, Rizio L, Zvijac JE, Uribe JW, Hechtman KS. Avulsion fracture of the ulnar sublime tubercle in overhead throwing athletes. *Am J Sports Med.* 2002;30(3):426-431.

31. Brown JH, Deluc SA. Growth plate injuries: Salter-Harris classification. *Am Fam Physician.* 1992;46:1180-1184.

32. Chen FS, Diaz VA, Loebenberg M, Rosen JE. Shoulder and elbow injuries in the skeletally immature athlete. *J Am Acad Orthop Surg.* 2005;13(3):172-185.

33. Lalonde KA, Letts M. Traumatic growth arrest of the distal tibia: a clinical and radiographic review. *Can J Surg.* 2005;48(2):143-147.

34. Vaquero J, Vidal C, Cubillo A. Intra-articular traumatic disorders of the knee in children and adolescents. *Clin Orthop.* 2005;(432):97-106.

35. Sartorelli KH, Vane DW. The diagnosis and management of children with blunt injury of the chest. *Semin Pediatr Surg.* 2004;13(2):98-105.

36. Bliss D, Silen M. Pediatric thoracic trauma. *Crit Care Med.* 2002;30(11 Suppl): S409-S415.

37. Neve V, Girard F, Flahault A, Boule M. Lung and thorax development during adolescence: relationship with pubertal status. *Eur Respir J.* 2002;20:1292-1298.

38. Goliath J, Mittal V, McDonough J. Traumatic handlebar hernia: a rare abdominal wall hernia. *J Pediatr Surg.* 2004;39(10):20-22.

39. Linuma Y, Yamazaki Y, Hirose Y, et al. A case of traumatic abdominal wall hernia that could not be identified until exploratory laparoscopy was performed. *Pediatr Surg Int.* 2005;21(1):54-57.

40. Mancel B, Aslam A. Traumatic abdominal wall hernia: an unusual bicycle handlebar injury. *Pediatr Surg Int.* 2003;19(11):746-747.

41. Erez I, Lazar L, Gutermacher M, Katz S. Abdominal injuries caused by bicycle handlebars. *Eur J Surg.* 2001;167(5):331-333.

42. Kubota A, Shono J, Yonekura T, et al. Handlebar hernia: case report and review of pediatric case. *Pediatr Surg Int.* 1999;15(5-6):411-412.

43. Nadler EP, Potoka DA, Shultz BL, Morrison KE, Ford HR, Gaines BA. The high morbidity associated with handlebar injuries in children. *J Trauma.* 2005;58(6):1171-1174.

44. Chen HY, Sheu MH, Tseng LM. Bicycle-handlebar hernia: a rare traumatic abdominal wall hernia. *J Chin Med Assoc.* 2005;68(6):283-285.

45. Radmayr C, Oswald J, Muller E, Holtl L, Bartsch G. Blunt renal trauma in children: 26 years clinical experience in an alpine region. *Eur Urol.* 2005;42(3):297-300.

46. Storsved JR, Rieger M. Acute kidney injury in a high school football player. *Journal of Athletic Training.* 2006;41(2 supplement):S74.

47. Patel DR, Shivdasani V, Baker RJ. Management of sports-related concussion in young athletes. *Sports Med.* 2005;35(8):671-684.

48. Rocchi G, Caroli E, Raco A, Salvati M, Delfini R. Traumatic epidural hematoma in children. *J Child Neurol.* 2005;20(7):569-572.

49. Broshek DK, Kaushik T, Freeman JR, Erlanger D, Webbe F, Barth JT. Sex differences in outcomes following sports-related concussion. *J Neurosurg.* 2005;102(5):856-863.

50. James Madison University Sports Medicine. Emergency action plan. Available at: http://www.jmusports.com/SupportServices/SportsMedicine/EmergencyActionPlan.asp. Accessed on July 3, 2006.

51. University of Georgia Sports Medicine. Information for visiting teams: emergency action plans. Accessed at http://georgiadogs.collegesports.com/sports-med/visiting-teams.html#track. Accessed on July 3, 2006.

Index

WAIT
...There's More!

SLACK Incorporated's Health Care Books and Journals offers a wide selection of products in the field of Athletic Training. We are dedicated to providing important works that educate, inform and improve the knowledge of our customers. Don't miss out on our other informative titles that will enhance your collection.

Special Tests for Orthopedic Examination, Third Edition
Jeff G. Konin, PhD, ATC, PT; Denise L. Wiksten, PhD, ATC; Jerome A. Isear, Jr., MS, PT, ATC-L; Holly Brader, MPH, RN, BSN, ATC
400 pp, Soft Cover, 2006, ISBN 10: 1-55642-741-7, ISBN 13: 978-1-55642-741-1, Order# 47417, **$38.95**

Special Tests for Orthopedic Examination has been used for 10 years by thousands of students, clinicians, and rehab professionals and is now available in a revised and updated third edition. Concise and pocket-sized, this handbook is an invaluable guide filled with the most current and practical clinical exam techniques used during an orthopedic examination. This *Third Edition* takes a user-friendly approach to visualizing and explaining more than 150 commonly used orthopedic special tests, including 11 new and modern tests.

Principles of Pharmacology for Athletic Trainers
Joel Houglum, PhD; Gary Harrelson, EdD, ATC; Deidre Leaver-Dunn, PhD, ATC
440 pp, Hard Cover, 2005, ISBN 10: 1-55642-594-5, ISBN 13: 978-1-55642-594-3, Order# 45945, **$44.95**

Principles of Pharmacology for Athletic Trainers is designed to help athletic training students understand the basic principles of pharmacology, as well as the broad classification of drugs. Drs. Joel Houglum, Gary Harrelson, and Deidre Leaver-Dunn have created a user-friendly format to help students meet the pharmacology domain outlined in the NATA Competencies in Athletic Training. Over 100 helpful figures and tables help to summarize the information presented and provide clinical examples.

Sports Emergency Care: A Team Approach
Robb Rehberg, PhD, ATC, NREMT
272 pp, Soft Cover, 2007, ISBN 10: 1-55642-798-0, ISBN 13: 978-1-55642-798-5, Order# 47980, **$42.95**

Athletic Training Exam Review: A Student Guide to Success, Third Edition
Lynn Van Ost, MEd, RN, PT, ATC; Karen Manfre, MA, ATR; Karen Lew, MEd, ATC, LAT
272 pp, Soft Cover, 2006, ISBN 10: 1-55642-764-6, ISBN 13: 978-1-55642-764-0, Order# 47646, **$42.95**

Clinical Skills Documentation Guide for Athletic Training, Second Edition
Herb Amato, DA, ATC; Christy D. Hawkins, ATC; Steven L. Cole, MEd, ATC, CSCS
464 pp, Soft Cover, 2006, ISBN 10: 1-55642-758-1, ISBN 13: 978-1-55642-758-9, Order# 47581, **$34.95**

Quick Reference Dictionary for Athletic Training, Second Edition
Julie N. Bernier, EdD, ATC
416 pp, Soft Cover, 2005, ISBN 10: 1-55642-666-6, ISBN 13: 978-1-55642-666-7, Order# 46666, **$29.95**

Athletic Training Student Primer: A Foundation for Success
Andrew P. Winterstein, PhD, ATC
256 pp, Soft Cover, 2003, ISBN 10: 1-55642-570-8, ISBN 13: 978-1-55642-570-7, Order# 45708, **$40.95**

Assessment of Nonorthopedic Sports Injuries: A Sideline Reference Manual
Jeff Lewandowski, DPT, SCS, ATC
176 pp, Soft Cover, 2000, ISBN 10: 1-55642-444-2, ISBN 13: 978-1-55642-444-1, Order# 44442, **$38.95**

Gait Analysis: Normal and Pathological Function
Jacquelin Perry, MD
556 pp, Hard Cover, 1992, ISBN 10: 1-55642-192-3, ISBN 13: 978-1-55642-192-1, Order# 11923, **$69.95**